Accidents Caused by Lightning Strikes

Fred Zack

Accidents Caused by Lightning Strikes

Medical Aspects

Springer

Fred Zack
Institut für Rechtsmedizin
Universität Rostock
Rostock, Deutschland

ISBN 978-3-662-71068-5 ISBN 978-3-662-71066-1 (eBook)
https://doi.org/10.1007/978-3-662-71066-1

Die Deutsche Nationalbibliothek verzeichnet diese Publikation in der Deutschen Nationalbibliografie; detaillierte bibliografische Daten sind im Internet über https://portal.dnb.de abrufbar.

Translation from the German language edition: "Unfälle durch Blitzschlag" by Fred Zack, © Der/die Herausgeber bzw. der/die Autor(en), exklusiv lizenziert an Springer-Verlag GmbH, DE, ein Teil von Springer Nature 2024. Published by Springer Berlin Heidelberg. All Rights Reserved.

This book is a translation of the original German edition "Unfälle durch Blitzschlag," 2nd edition, by Fred Zack, published by Springer-Verlag GmbH, DE in 2024. The translation was done with the help of an artificial intelligence machine translation tool. A subsequent human revision was done primarily in terms of content, so that the book will read stylistically differently from a conventional translation. Springer Nature works continuously to further the development of tools for the production of books and on the related technologies to support the authors.

This Springer imprint is published by the registered company Springer-Verlag GmbH, DE, part of Springer Nature.
The registered company address is: Heidelberger Platz 3, 14197 Berlin, Germany

For my wife Sabine, my daughter Tabea, and my grandchildren Elmar and Marla

Foreword

Accidents caused by lightning strikes are more common than generally assumed and yet a topic that has not been sufficiently addressed for years. The extremely knowledgeable, linguistically precise, and well-structured book by the forensic scientist Fred Zack combines medical knowledge against the backdrop of meteorological and electrical engineering facts as well as legal aspects.

A retrospective with competently selected quotes from the literature on the investigation of lightning accidents is supplemented by the presentation of emergency medical measures and clinical diagnostics in the case of lightning strike victims who survive. The wide spectrum of health consequences of lightning strikes is impressively explained using examples. This is supplemented by the external and internal post-mortem examination findings, knowledge of which can be expected from forensic doctors and pathologists, but which also represents important background knowledge for other medical disciplines. The statements are rounded off with a literature list related to each chapter, illustrations, and tables.

This provides all readers—for the first time in decades—with a new, current, fact-rich book that closes more than one knowledge gap. A work, indispensable for the technical and medical assessment by experts, a work that deserves wider distribution beyond specialized circles.

Gießen, Germany
in the summer of 2023

Reinhard Dettmeyer

Preface

For decades, the number of fatal lightning strike accidents involving people living in Germany or other developed nations has been declining.

Why then a book about lightning strike accidents from a medical perspective?

- Because the observed decline in the number of fatal lightning accidents does not say anything about the number of surviving victims who can develop both early and late health consequences of a lightning strike.
- Because the last specialist book on this topic in Germany appeared more than 60 years ago and only from the perspective of the disciplines of neurology and psychiatry.
- Because numerous victims of a lightning strike accident, who are organized, for example, in the international society "Lightning Strike & Electric Shock Survivors International" (LS&ESSI, Inc.) founded in the USA, complain about a lack of medical expertise in diagnosis and therapy, especially of late damage.
- Because the specialist knowledge is obviously incomplete even among experienced forensic doctors, who are probably the most likely to come into contact with this topic in their professional lives.
- Because the numerous surviving and killed victims of lightning strikes in the developing countries of the world make the topic still current—also taking into account global mobility and the international activities of medical aid organizations.

When I presented my first lethal lightning accident at the 75th annual meeting of the German Society for Forensic Medicine in 1996 in Zurich—it was a 27-year-old man who died 5 days after the accident and showed an acute lightning traumatic myocardial necrosis—an experienced senior physician asked me what the man's coronary arteries looked like. "Without pathological findings," I replied. "I don't believe you," he retorted. My colleague had never heard that myocardial infarction-like findings can follow immediately after a lightning accident, regardless of the coronary status.

In my further professional life, this was not the only case in which experienced forensic doctors revealed gaps in their specialist knowledge about lightning strike accidents in personal conversations.

For the reasons mentioned, the present specialist book on lightning strike injuries was created, which includes numerous aspects of this extraordinary type of accident from an interdisciplinary human medical perspective.

Rostock, Germany
in the summer of 2023

Fred Zack

Acknowledgments

My thanks go to:

Andreas Büttner for his tireless support of my entire scientific activity, not only in the field of lightning research,

Ryan Blumenthal, Michael Rock, and Reinhard Dettmeyer for their specialized support in clarifying specific questions,

Charlotte Börngen for her creative suggestions and support in the creation of numerous illustrations,

Larissa Bremer for her participation in the evaluation of accidents caused by lightning strikes,

Sabine Gadewoll for her support in the evaluation of statistical surveys,

Anna Kraetz and Meenakshi Rajenthiran from Springer Nature Publishing for their patience and effort in the development and completion of the book and

"Last, but not least," I thank my family, especially Sabine, Tabea, Tobias, Elmar, and Marla, who have endured my absence with patience and great understanding.

Rostock
in the summer of 2023

Fred Zack

Contents

Abbreviations

ABB	Committee for Lightning Protection and Lightning Research
AV-Block	Atrioventricular Block
AWMF	Association of the Scientific Medical Societies e. V.
CAB	Chromotrope Aniline Blue Staining
CK	Creatine Kinase
CK-MB	Creatine Kinase—Isoenzyme Cardiac Muscle
CK-MM	Creatine Kinase—Isoenzyme Skeletal Muscle
CRPS	Complex Regional Pain Syndrome, Ger. komplexes regionales Schmerzsyndrom
CT	Computer Tomogram
EEG	Electroencephalogram
ECG	Electrocardiogram
EMG	Electromyography
ENG	Electroneurography
GOT	Glutamate Oxaloacetate Transaminase
HE	Hematoxylin-Eosin Staining
HNO	Ear-Nose-Throat
ICD	International Statistical Classification of Diseases and Related Health Problems, i.e., international classification of diseases
MRT	Magnetic Resonance Tomogram
PKW	Passenger car
QST	Quantitative Sensory Testing
ROSC	Return of Spontaneous Circulation, Ger. Restoration of a Spontaneous Circulation
SSR	Sympathetic Skin Response, eng. sympathetic skin reaction
USA	United States of America
UV	Ultraviolet
VDE	Association of Electrical Engineering, Electronics, Information Technology e. V.

List of Figures

List of Tables

1 Introduction

At any given time, there are about 2000 thunderstorms on our planet. Based on ground and satellite measurements, it is estimated that between 30 and 100 lightning strikes occur on Earth every second. Over the course of a day, there can be up to 9 million lightning strikes on the globe (Uman 2008). The geographical distribution of lightning is not homogeneous. The frequency of thunderstorms decreases continuously from the equator to the polar regions (Heidler and Stimper 2009).

Most lightning strikes on Earth occur over land, as the warming of the land by the sun is the most common source of the rising heated moist air needed to generate opposite charges within a cloud. In general, the hotter and more humid the local atmosphere, the more thunderstorms and lightning occur (see Chap. 3).

In parts of tropical Africa and Indonesia, more than 200 thunderstorm days occur in some places each year. On the coasts of Oregon and Washington in the United States of America (USA), there are virtually no lightning strikes, as the Pacific Ocean keeps the air cool and suppresses the upward movement of air. In contrast, the central and southwestern parts of Florida, which have the highest number of lightning strikes per square kilometer in the USA in most years, have thunderstorms on about 90 days per year.

For the Federal Republic of Germany, there are no available statistical frequencies of lightning strikes per square kilometer and unit of time. In a statistic for the year 2016, based on the total area of the federal states, the most thunderstorm days occurred in Bavaria with 131, followed by Baden-Württemberg with 123 days (UBIMET 2017).

Lightning strikes can harm people and their habitats in various ways. For example, the lightning of a thunderstorm can harm people's health or cause their death. In the case of primary energy transfer mechanisms, there are accidents with injuries to individual people or even groups of people (see Chap. 4). However, if a lightning strike ignites a large fire, triggers an explosion, or causes a plane crash, there can also be secondary damages, which can have very high casualty numbers. For example, on August 18, 1769,

F. Zack, *Accidents Caused by Lightning Strikes*,
https://doi.org/10.1007/978-3-662-71066-1_1

a lightning strike hit the San Nazaro bastion in Brescia, Northern Italy, igniting a fire that detonated about 90,000 kg of gunpowder stored there, leading to a disastrous explosion. Huge chunks of rock were hurled at people, houses, and churches within a radius of about one kilometer. This lightning-induced explosion killed about 3000 people and destroyed a sixth of the city (Uman 2008). Reports also exist of crashes of large airplanes, following lightning-induced explosions of the tanks, with the death of all persons on board in 1959 in Italy (near Milan) and 1963 in the USA (Maryland) (Uman 1986).

Furthermore, lightning strikes can cause great damage to man-made community objects. For example, on the early evening of July 13, 1977, lightning struck several 345,000-V transmission lines located about 30 miles north of New York City, which supplied the greater area of this city with electricity. This was followed by a chain reaction of electrical events, resulting in the entire city being cut off from the power supply at 9:34 PM. It took about 24 hours to restore the electricity supply. Approximately 9 million people spent a night and a day without electricity. By the end of the power outage, nearly 2000 stores had been looted or damaged and more than 3500 people had been arrested. The cost of this lightning-induced power outage was estimated at about 350 million US dollars (Sugarman 1978).

Thunderstorms with cloud-to-ground lightning can also cause great damage to the plant and animal kingdom. For example, lightning-induced fires burned about 320,000 hectares, i.e., 36% of the area of the world's first national park, along with countless animals and plants, during a dry summer in 1988 in Yellowstone National Park, USA. About 25,000 people fought against numerous fires until the first snowfall of the winter. In total, approximately 150 million US dollars were spent on firefighting (Renkin and Despain 1992; Uman 2008).

Due to the relatively rare occurrence of lightning accidents involving personal injury and the severely limited possibilities of replicating such events in animal experiments, the investigation of human injuries after a lightning strike is still fraught with problems to this day. The current expert knowledge about the health consequences of lightning accidents for humans predominantly comes from retrospective analyses of individual accidents or from studies in which several such accidents were evaluated. Therefore, the current medical lightning research, unlike numerous other research areas in human medicine, covers a relatively large time frame. However, a significant development is noticeable in recent decades. While in the last century many physicians presented their research results for their field as sole authors (Cooper 1980; Jellinek 1903; Krauland 1951; Panse 1925; Peters 1983; Wetli 1996), there were subsequently increasing publications by author teams from different medical disciplines (Andrews et al. 1989; Cherington et al. 1998, 2001; Cooray et al. 2007; Jonas et al. 2002; Ritenour et al. 2008; Tadler et al. 2017; Zack et al. 1997).

In recent years, there has been a trend for physicians to increasingly cooperate with scientists from non-medical disciplines, such as electrical engineers, meteorologists, or statisticians, and to publish their results together. This approach can only be welcomed for the analysis of lightning accidents involving people, as it is expected that this interdisciplinary cooperation will lead to a better understanding of the accidents and their consequences for people's health (Cooper and Holle 2019; Cooper et al. 2017; Hunt et al. 2020; Navarrete-Aldana et al. 2014; Zack et al. 2013).

References

Andrews CJ, Darveniza M, Mackerras D (1989) Lightning injury a review of clinical aspects, pathophysiology and treatment. Adv Trauma 4:241–252

Cherington M, Wachtel H, Yarnell PR (1998) Could lightning injury be magnetically induced? Lancet 351:1788

Cherington M, Kurtzman R, Krider EP, Yarnell PR (2001) Mountain medical mystery. Unwitnessed death of a healthy young man, caused by lightning. Am J Forensic Med Pathol 22:296–298

Cooper MA (1980) Lightning injuries: prognostic signs for death. Ann Emerg Med 9:134–138

Cooper MA, Holle RL (2019) Reducing lightning injuries worldwide. Springer, Cham

Cooper MA, Andrews CJ, Holle RL, Blumenthal R, Navarette-Aldana N (2017) Lightning-related injuries and safety. In: Auerbach P, Cushing T, Harris N (Hrsg) Auerbach's wilderness medicine. 7. Aufl. Elsevier, Philadelphia, S 71–117

Cooray V, Cooray C, Andrews CJ (2007) Lightning caused injuries in humans. J Electrostatics 65:386–394

Heidler F, Stimper K (2009) Blitz und Blitzschutz. VDE, Berlin Offenbach

Hunt HGP, Blumenthal R, Nixon KJ, Gomes C (2020) A multidisciplinary forensic analysis of two lightning deaths observed in South Africa. Int J Disaster Risk Reduct 51:101814

Jellinek S (1903) Elektropathologie: Die Erkrankungen durch Blitzschlag und elektrischen Starkstrom in klinischer und forensischer Darstellung. Enke, Stuttgart

Jonas L, Fulda G, Nizze H, Zimmermann R, Gross G, Zack F, Kröning G, Holzhüter G, Haas HJ (2002) Detection of gold particles in the neck skin after lightning stroke with evaporation of an ornamental chain. Ultrastruct Pathol 26:153–159

Krauland W (1951) Schäden und Todesfälle durch Blitzschlag. Dtsch Zeitschr Gerichtl Med 40:298–312

Navarrete-Aldana N, Cooper MA, Holle RL (2014) Lightning fatalities in Colombia from 2000 to 2009. Nat Hazards 74:1349–1362

Panse F (1925) Über Schädigungen des Nervensystems durch Blitzschlag. Mschr Psychiat Neurol 59:323–338

Peters WJ (1983) Lightning injury. Can Med Assoc J 128:148–150

Renkin RA, Despain DG (1992) Fuel moisture, forest type, and lightning caused fire in Yellowstone National Park. Can J Forest Res 22:37–45

Ritenour AE, Morton MJ, McManus JG, Barillo DJ, Cancio LC (2008) Lightning injury: a review. Burns 34:585–594

Sugarman R (1978) New York City's blackout: a $350 million drain. IEEE Spectr 15:44–46

Tadler M, Rüegg E, Niquille M, Gencer B, Gautschi OP, Pittet-Cuénod MA (2017) Multi-organ injuries due to a lightning strike: a case report highlighting the importance of a multi-disciplinary approach. Case Reports Plast Surg Hand Surg 4:1–4

UBIMET (2017) Blitzdatenreport Deutschland 2016. https://www.ubimet.com/blitzdatenreport-deutschland-2016/Zugegriffen. Accessed: 22 Febr 2023

Uman MA (1986) All about lightning. Dover Publications, New York

Uman MA (2008) The art and science of lightning protection. Cambridge University Press, Cambridge New York Melbourne Madrid Kapstadt Singapur Sao Paulo Delhi

Wetli CV (1996) Keraunopathology. An analysis of 45 fatalities. Am J Forensic Med Pathol 17:89–98

Zack F, Hammer U, Klett I, Wegener R (1997) Myocardial injury due to lightning. Int J Legal Med 110:326–328

Zack F, Raphael T, Kupfer J, Jokuszies A, Vogt PM, Büttner A, Püschel K, Schalke B, Todt M, Dettmeyer R (2013) Vier Todesopfer nach einem Blitzunfall auf einem Golfplatz. Rechtsmedizin 23:114–118

Historical

2

The weather phenomena of thunderstorms, lightning, and thunder have always instilled fear and terror in humanity. In ancient Greece, lightning was considered an expression of the wrath of the god Zeus (Ravitch et al. 1961). In contrast, among the ancient Germans, there was also the widespread belief that thunderstorms were associated with the restoration of justice and peace. The extraordinarily powerful god Donar was believed to have protected people from attacks by hostile monsters by striking them down with a stone throwing axe, which he hurled away with a lightning bolt (Golther 2003). Furthermore, numerous peoples revered the ground struck by lightning and subsequently considered it sacred (Cooper 1980).

In the middle of the 18th century, humanity's view of the natural phenomenon of thunderstorms began to change. A significant contribution to this was made by the American Benjamin Franklin, who, with his life-threatening experiments with a prepared flying kite during thunderstorm conditions between 1746–1753, was able to prove that thunderbolts are natural electrical discharges (Uman 1986).

The history of the medical findings recorded in German-language literature and still available today in cases of lightning accidents with injuries to persons dates back to an event on June 25, 1785, and is particularly the history of Lichtenberg figures. According to the Royal Privy Councillor and personal physician Mayer, on this day a lightning bolt struck the Gubener gate guard in Frankfurt an der Oder, damaged the building, and injured four soldiers sitting on a bench in front of the guard. Subsequently, illustrations of the findings of two accident victims were produced by the Lithographic Institute of Kraatz in Berlin. Privy Councillor Mayer (1795) described in the *New Remarks and Experiences for the Enrichment of Wound Surgery and Medical Knowledge* published by Theden: "*Among the remarkable phenomena produced by the movement of electrical matter, electrical figures, or as others call them, electrical flowers, which form on the electrophorus invented by Volta, certainly deserve our admiration.*" Mayer may not have

F. Zack, *Accidents Caused by Lightning Strikes*,
https://doi.org/10.1007/978-3-662-71066-1_2

been aware of the results of the experiments of the German physicist Lichtenberg from 1777, otherwise he would probably have been the first to establish a connection between the star-shaped patterns in the dust of an insulating plate of Lichtenberg's electrophorus and the findings observed in 1785 on the two lightning victims in Frankfurt an der Oder.

This association was reserved for the Kiel physician Pfaffe (1825), who wrote in *Gehler's Physical Dictionary* under the article "Lightning": *"Remarkable are the drawings, which the lightning sometimes leaves on the skin, completely corresponding with the Lichtenberg figures on the electrophorus. Brandis ... tells of such a case where spots the size of a guilder, white in the middle and radiating ramifications around, were shown on the chest of a woman killed by lightning."*

In the middle of the 19th century, the Frankfurt physician Stricker (1861, 1863, 1872) began as the first doctor in the German-speaking area to collect and evaluate case reports on lightning accidents with personal injuries (Figs. 2.1 and 2.2). Given the lack of scientific publications at that time and his great interest in the topic, it is not surprising that 78 years later he also extensively revisited the lightning accident of the soldiers of the Gubener Torwache. In this context, Stricker described, referring to Mayer, that at least one victim showed burnt hair and blistered skin in addition to the electrical figures. Regarding the now more frequently described Lichtenberg figures in lightning victims, Stricker, supported by the Berliner Langerhans (1862), held the view that these were caused by the injection of tree-like branched blood vessels of the skin (Stricker 1861). This was contradicted by the prosector of pathology in Zurich, Rindfleisch (1862), as he had examined a man killed by lightning and his results spoke against the hypothesis of Stricker and Langerhans. The erythema identified by Rindfleisch did not anatomically match blood vessel courses. Moreover, he was the first to describe an interrupted erythema, caused by skin folds due to wearing a *"tightly fastened leather belt"*. By the middle of the 19th century, numerous findings were already known in victims of lightning accidents, such as torn or perforated clothing, melted metal pieces, singed hair, band-like burns, tree-like figures on the skin, wounds under the feet or black discoloration of the neck when wearing a necklace. In surviving victims, symptoms and damages such as loss of consciousness, burning pain, convulsive muscle twitching, fatigue, weakness, sensitivity, oppression, accelerated pulse, and stiffness of the limbs were described. The disappearance of the branches on the skin was also mentioned (Stricker 1872). As therapy, bloodletting was performed on people who had survived a lightning accident.

On the other hand, Stricker (1861, 1872) critically dealt with the following statements of the French physician Boudin: *"Sometimes lightning kills, sometimes it heals. Here it causes loss of sight, hearing, movement, there it heals a paralytic, a deaf person, a blind person. It undresses its victims, destroys the clothes and spares the body or it destroys the corpse and spares the clothes. Here it kills suddenly, on the spot, so that the dead person remains upright, sitting or riding, there on the other hand the struck person is hurled 20 m away and one finds him in the foliage of chestnut trees."* (Stricker 1861). Stricker, in his extensive collection for the time (27 lightning accidents with personal

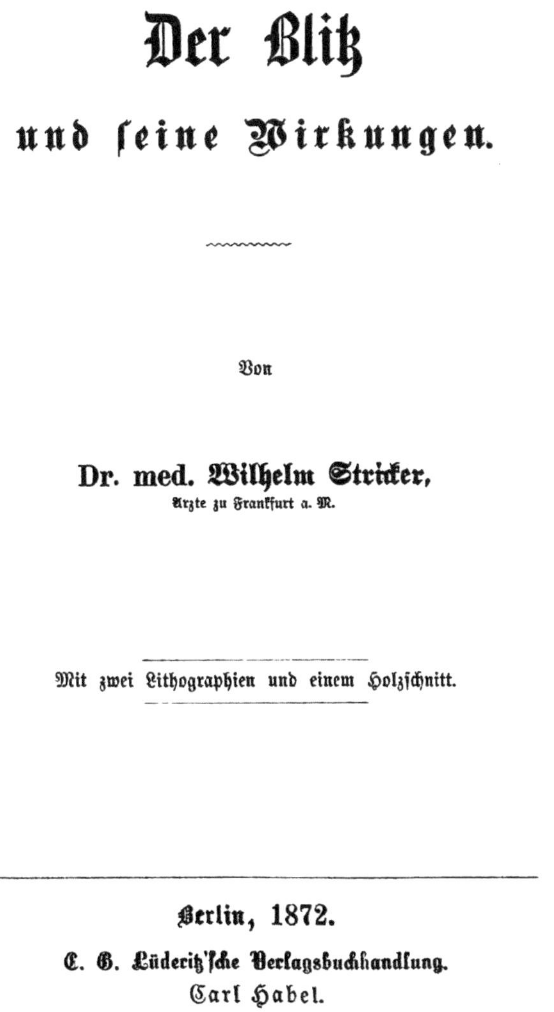
Der Blitz

und seine Wirkungen.

Von

Dr. med. Wilhelm Stricker,
Arzte zu Frankfurt a. M.

Mit zwei Lithographien und einem Holzschnitt.

Berlin, 1872.
C. G. Lüderitz'sche Verlagsbuchhandlung.
Carl Habel.

Fig. 2.1 Title page of the first German-language book on injuries caused by lightning strike by Wilhelm Stricker. (Stricker 1872)

injuries from the professional literature), could *"not find any authenticated report"* of healed blindness or deafness and referred the *"healing power of lightning to the realm of fables"*.

Nearly 20 years later, in 1891, a lightning accident was reported near Tübingen, resulting in 2 deaths and 18 injured persons. The special feature of the publication is that it contains the *"section protocol on the person killed by lightning on August 15, 1888 … from Pfrondorf, 27 years old, 24 h after death"*. The main finding is described by the pathologist as follows: *"On the right … at the rib pillar edge and slightly downwards crossing it in a longitudinal extension of 11 cm and a transverse extension of 5 cm, a pale violet, not raised blotchy discoloration of the skin, which disappears under finger*

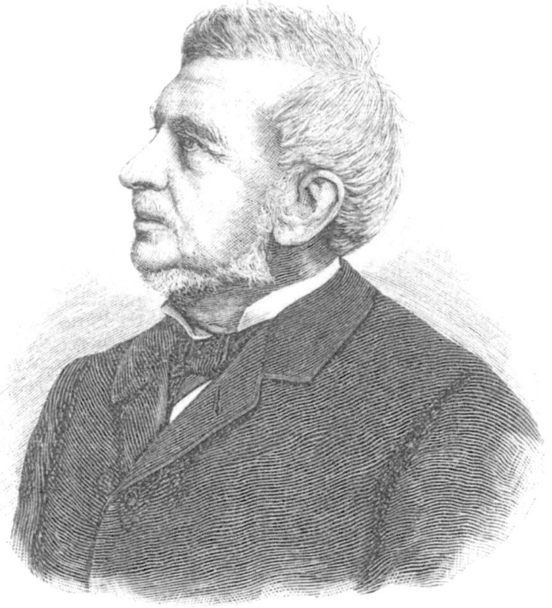

Fig. 2.2 Wilhelm Stricker on January 1, 1892. (From the Tripota database in the Scientific Library of the City of Trier/City Archive, author unknown)

pressure. The discoloration consists of spots, but especially of stripes, which appear clearly tree-like branched, or also resemble the appearance of a coarse coral tree … Nothing special to see when cutting in." The summary: "*The result of the autopsy is hardly suitable to give an explanation of the sudden death*" reveals a certain helplessness of the pathologist (Ebertz 1891). Almost simultaneously, the Viennese forensic pathologist Haberda (1891) agreed with Rindfleisch's view on the pathogenesis of lightning figures: "*The redness also decidedly does not adhere to certain branches of a vessel, thus does not represent an injection of this vessel, but belongs to various neighboring areas and its branched arrangement can only be related to the way the lightning moves on the surface and radiates sideways.*"

At the beginning of the 20th century, Jellinek's (1903) textbook *Electropathology: Diseases caused by lightning and high voltage electricity in clinical and forensic representation* was published in Stuttgart, a milestone in the history of medical examinations of lightning and electricity victims. The fact that Jellinek's work was of considerable relevance is also demonstrated by the fact that the edition that can currently be purchased in 2024 is a reproduction of the original work and bears the stamp of the "Boston Medical Library" with the date "Mar 21 1904" (Fig. 2.3). Several examples prove how valuable Jellinek's results published 120 years ago still are for medicine today. On the one hand, he considered the long-known Lichtenberg figures as pathognomonic for a lightning strike. On the other hand, Jellinek also classified the singed body hair found after

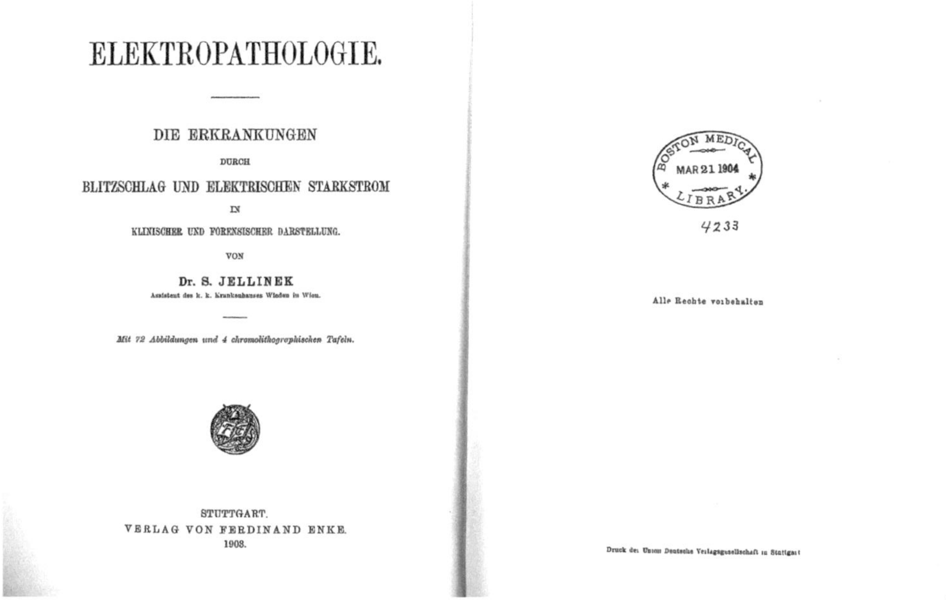

ELEKTROPATHOLOGIE.

DIE ERKRANKUNGEN
DURCH
BLITZSCHLAG UND ELEKTRISCHEN STARKSTROM
IN
KLINISCHER UND FORENSISCHER DARSTELLUNG.
VON
Dr. S. JELLINEK
Assistent des k. k. Krankenhauses Wieden in Wien.

Mit 72 Abbildungen und 4 chromolithographischen Tafeln.

STUTTGART.
VERLAG VON FERDINAND ENKE.
1903.

Druck der Union Deutsche Verlagsgesellschaft in Stuttgart

Fig. 2.3 Stefan Jellinek's milestone *Electropathology* with a stamp from the "Boston Medical Library" dated March 21, 1904. (Jellinek 1903)

lightning strikes as a very characteristic finding. With this knowledge on the day of the autopsy in August 1888, the pathologist of the lightning victim from Pfrondorf would certainly have had an explanation for the *"sudden death"* of the 27-year-old woman. Furthermore, Jellinek already pointed out the possibility of a traceless or trace-free homicide by electric current.

The state of medical knowledge at the beginning of the previous century was summarized under the keyword "lightning strike" in Platen's *The New Healing Method. Textbook of natural lifestyle, health care and natural healing method*(Fig. 2.4). It also contains numerous hints for the treatment of lightning strike victims, such as moving to a cool place, letting them smell ammonia, pouring water over them, or burying the completely undressed victim 2-3 feet deep with the head raised at the scene of the accident (Platen 1913).

Two decades later, Nippe (1932) from Königsberg in Prussia took up the topic of Lichtenberg figures again in the form of histological examinations. He found uncharacteristic findings such as epithelial lesions and hyperemia of the skin capillaries.

From Innsbruck, the forensic pathologist Krauland, who had just moved to Münster, reported on 3 lightning accidents, 2 of which were fatal (1951). In the case of a deceased 16-year-old girl who was picking cherries in a tree, exceptionally large skin burns were found on her chest and abdomen. Since all 3 lightning victims showed characteristic

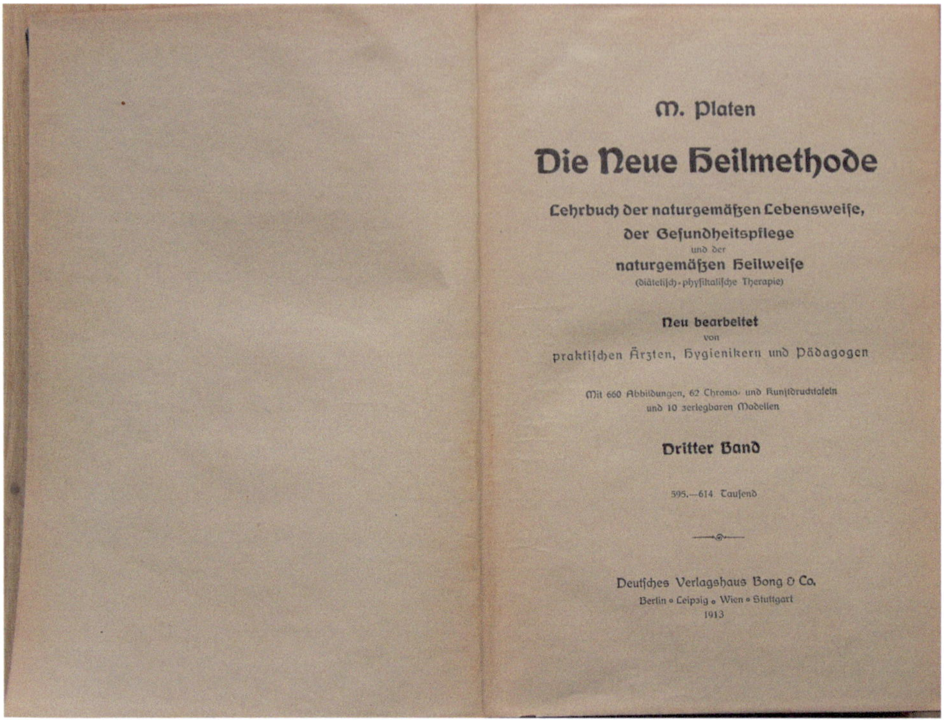

M. Platen

Die Neue Heilmethode

Lehrbuch der naturgemäßen Lebensweise,
der Gesundheitspflege
und der
naturgemäßen Heilweise
(diätetisch-physikalische Therapie)

Neu bearbeitet
von
praktischen Ärzten, Hygienikern und Pädagogen

Mit 660 Abbildungen, 62 Chromo- und Kunstdrucktafeln
und 10 zerlegbaren Modellen

Dritter Band

595.—614. Tausend

Deutsches Verlagshaus Bong & Co.
Berlin • Leipzig • Wien • Stuttgart
1913

Fig. 2.4 In Platen's *The New Healing Method*, it was recommended as initial treatment that victims of a lightning strike should be buried in the earth, with the exception of the head. (Platen 1913)

findings after the accidents, he expressed doubts about the existence of lightning accidents in which no characteristic findings would have been detectable on the victim. Later case reports showed that Krauland's concerns were unfounded (Khartade et al. 2023; Wetli 1996). The textbooks of forensic medicine/legal medicine, which appeared at irregular intervals, contained not only summarizing presentations on the topic but also extraordinary individual cases. Thus, Mueller (1953) from Heidelberg described the consequences of lightning accidents under the heading "Cosmic Electricity" and reported on a lightning accident from Bremen, where the homicide squad had initially investigated due to the location of the discovery, a street in the city. The field of Forensic Medicine was supported in the research and increase of knowledge of the effects of electrical current, including lightning strikes, by numerous other disciplines of human medicine. The publication of the work *Clinical Electropathology* by the internist Koeppen from Wolfsburg and the neurologist and psychiatrist Panse from Bonn was another milestone in the history of medical examinations of victims of a lightning or electrical accident. In particular, the lightning accident of April 13, 1925 at the Königstein Fortress with 29 victims is described in detail (Panse 1925, 1955). Numerous forensic publications subsequently drew on the interdisciplinary knowledge compiled by Koeppen and Panse. Herold (1960) from Leipzig criticized in the *Textbook of Forensic Medicine* edited by Prokop the term *"cosmic electricity"* and emphasized that the atmospheric electrical discharge processes accompanying a thunderstorm, which impress visually and acoustically as lightning, are of *"terrestrial nature"*.

Even though Iranyi et al. (1962) were from Budapest, the medical community in the German-speaking world took great interest in the results on the acute symptoms in survivors of 156 lightning accidents from Hungary, which were published in the Munich Medical Weekly (Radam 1975). Weimann and Prokop (1963) showed for the first time in an *Atlas of Forensic Medicine* a Lichtenberg figure on the shoe of a man who had been killed by a lightning strike. In addition to the finding, the nomenclature *"Lichtenstein's lightning figure"* was remarkable.

Koeppen (1965) once again contributed with a review on personal injuries caused by lightning and 9 case presentations. It is astonishing in retrospect that even the 3rd edition of the *Textbook of Forensic Medicine for Physicians and Lawyers* by Ponsold (1967) from Münster, which comprised 645 pages, did not contain any contribution on lightning accidents. This disregard is also remarkable against the background that there had been up to 100 deaths per year in Germany after 1950 (Harms 1956; Koeppen 1965; Schniers 2005).

In contrast to the aforementioned textbook by Ponsold, Sellier (1975) described the consequences of lightning impacts over 4 pages in the 2nd edition of Mueller's *Forensic Medicine*. He also described an extraordinary accident in which a field worker had died during working hours. The responsible professional association ordered an autopsy, which was carried out in an institute for pathology. The autopsy, which took place 3 days after the event, revealed advanced post-mortem changes. The pathologist noted a diagnosis of cardiac death. As a result, the professional association refused to pay an accident pension. The wife, who was near the accident site at the time of the accident and had chosen a different shelter from the storm than her husband, claimed in all instances that her husband had been struck by lightning. Four years after the event, the man's clothing, which the wife had kept, was examined by an experienced forensic pathologist. He found characteristic signs of a lightning strike in the form of tears in the trousers and a sock, as well as the perforation of the upper material of a leather shoe. After submitting his report, the widow was granted the accident pension.

Sellier (1975) concluded from this that in case of a suspicion of death by lightning strike, the victim's clothing should be carefully inspected, as it may provide the only clue for the correct diagnosis. This view was also supported by Schaidt (1977) with his publication "*Traces on clothing in the event of a lightning accident*". In this work, he described an accident in which a 63-year-old man was found dead under an oak tree in a forest in Nuremberg-Langwasser on August 12, 1975. Next to him lay his also lifeless German Shepherd. The initial considerations included that the dog should or could have caused the observed damage to the man's clothing. No autopsy was performed.

Another medical lightning researcher who significantly contributed to today's interdisciplinary expertise with his experiments and literature research is the Viennese doctor Karobath (1977). In particular, his contribution to the pathophysiology of the death mechanism by lightning strike from a clinical perspective was and is of considerable relevance not only for forensic medicine.

In the period after the case from Nuremberg-Langwasser by Schaidt (1977), rare findings after lightning accidents were repeatedly published in the history of forensic medicine based solely on autopsy results. One reason for this is certainly that findings from the external autopsy in the case of death by lightning strike are more diagnostic than the results of the internal autopsy (Zack and Büttner 2020b). Another cause lies in the trend observed for many years of a decrease in official autopsy orders, at least in the Federal Republic of Germany (Madea and Weckbecker 2020). The number of publications on lethal lightning accidents without performed autopsies has increased in the recent history of forensic medicine (König and Pedal 1982; Püschel et al. 2009; Zack et al. 2010, 2013).

After Nippe (1932) and Krauland (1951) focused their histological examinations of lightning victims on the Lichtenberg figures of the skin, the spectrum of examined organs and tissues was expanded with subsequent publications and, in addition to the skin, particularly affected the myocardium (Dettmeyer 2018; Janssen 1977; Möhle et al. 2015; Pollak et al. 1988; Zack et al. 1997).

Pollak (2000) addressed problems with diagnosis in his publication "*Misrecognition of fatal high-voltage and lightning accidents*". Like Sellier (1975) before him, he reported that characteristic, albeit sometimes only slightly pronounced, findings after a lightning strike were overlooked or misinterpreted during the medical autopsy at the accident site. Pollak concluded from this that a holistic inclusion of the discovery situation, the clothing findings, and the autopsy of the entire body surface are necessary for the correct diagnosis.

Even though the number of lethal lightning accidents in the leading industrial countries has significantly decreased in recent decades, the professional interest in this rare type of injury and cause of death, as numerous current publications in professional journals and books show, has by no means decreased (Blumenthal et al. 2022; Cooper and Holle 2019; Gomes 2021; Zack and Büttner 2020a, b). The accumulated expertise of the last 150 years should not be disregarded due to the decreased number of cases in many countries, but should be considered with due critical restraint (Medvei 1975).

References

Blumenthal R, Noxon KJ, Gomes C, Hunt HGP (2022) Lightning metallization injury. Am J Forensic Med Pathol 43:e93–e95

Cooper MA (1980) Lightning injuries: prognostics signs for death. Ann Emerg Med 9:134–138

Cooper MA, Holle RL (2019) Reducing lightning injuries worldwide. Springer, Cham

Dettmeyer RB (2018) Forensic Histopathology. Fundamentals and Perspectives. Springer, Heidelberg
Ebertz M (1891) Ueber Blitzverletzungen. Dtsch Med Wochenschr 36:1048–1051
Golther W (2003) Handbuch der Germanischen Mythologie. Fourier, Wiesbaden
Gomes C (2021) Lightning. Science, engineering, and economic implications for developing countries. Springer, Singapore
Haberda A (1891) Ein Fall von Tötung durch Blitzschlag. Wien Klin Wochenschr 82:588
Harms W (1956) Personenblitzschäden. Elektromedizin 1:153–158
Herold K (1960) Der Elektrotod. In: Prokop O (Eds) Lehrbuch der gerichtlichen Medizin. Volk und Gesundheit, Berlin, pp 127–141
Iranyi J, Orovecz B, Somogyi E, Iranyi K (1962) Das Blitztrauma in neuer Sicht. Münch Med Wochenschr 104:1496–1500
Janssen W (1977) Forensische Histologie. Schmidt-Römhild, Lübeck
Jellinek S (1903) Elektropathologie: Die Erkrankungen durch Blitzschlag und elektrischen Starkstrom in klinischer und forensischer Darstellung. Enke, Stuttgart
Karobath H, Redtenbacher M, Hofecker G, Walde I, Syré G (1977) Zur Frage der Todesursache beim Blitzunfall. Münch Med Wochenschr 119:29–32
Khartade HK, Shrivastava S, Vashisht J, Phukan A, Palazhy PP, Meshram VP (2023) Delayed death due to lightning: an autopsy case report highlighting diagnostic and medicolegal issues. J Burn Care Res 44:996–999
König HG, Pedal I (1982) Analyse eines Blitzunfalls. In: Barz J, Bösche J, Frohberg H, Joachim H, Käppner R, Mattern R (Eds) Fortschritte der Rechtsmedizin. Springer, Berlin Heidelberg New York, pp 77–88
Koeppen S (1965) Personenschäden durch Blitzeinwirkung. Med Klin 60:1390–1393
Krauland W (1951) Schäden und Todesfälle durch Blitzschlag. Dtsch Z Gerichtl Med 40:298–312
Langerhans P (1862) Zwei Fälle von Blitzschlag. Arch Path Anat Physiol Klin Med 24:200–201
Madea B, Weckbecker K (2020) Todesfeststellung und Leichenschau für Hausärzte. Springer, Berlin
Mayer R (1795) Neue Bemerkungen und Erfahrungen zur Wundarzneikunst und Arzneigelahrtheit. III. Theil, Berlin, pp 166
Medvei VC (1975) Lightning. Br Med J 1:208
Möhle F, Preuss J, Madea B, Doberentz E (2015) Vier Tage überlebter Blitzschlag nach zunächst erfolgreicher Reanimation. Rechtsmedizin 25:561–565
Mueller B (1953) Gerichtliche Medizin. Springer, Berlin Göttingen Heidelberg
Nippe M (1932) Zur Genese und Histologie von Blitzfiguren und elektrischen Strommarken. Virchows Arch 285:1–11
Panse F (1925) Über Schädigungen des Nervensystems durch Blitzschlag. Mschr Psychiat Neurol 59:323–338
Panse F (1955) Die Neurologie des elektrischen Unfalls und des Blitzschlags. In: Koeppen S, Panse F (Eds) Klinische Elektropathologie. Thieme, Stuttgart, pp 139–414
Pfaffe M (1825) Blitz. In: Gehler JST (Hrsg) Gehlers physikalisches Wörterbuch. Schwickert, Leipzig, pp 1016
Platen M (1913) Die neue Heilmethode. Bd 1. Deutsches Verlagshaus Bong & Co, Berlin Leipzig Wien Stuttgart
Pollak S (2000) Verkennung von tödlichen Hochspannungs- und Blitzunfällen. Arch Kriminol 206:168–179
Pollak S, Stellwag-Carion C, Binder R (1988) Zur Pathomorphologie tödlicher Blitzunfälle. In: Bauer G (Hrsg) Gerichtsmedizin – Festschrift für Wilhelm Holczabek. Deuticke, Wien, pp 139–153

Ponsold A (1967) Lehrbuch der Gerichtlichen Medizin, 3rd edn. Thieme, Stuttgart
Püschel K, Kalka R, Schulz F, Zack F (2009) Tod durch Blitzschlag. Fahrrad als „(Faraday'sche) Falle". Rechtsmedizin 19:102–104
Radam G, Strauch H (1975) Der Blitzschlag. In: Prokop O, Göhler W (eds) Forensische Medizin. 3rd edn. Volk und Gesundheit, Berlin, pp 163–164
Ravitch MM, Lane R, Safar P (1961) Lightning stroke: report of a case with recovery after cardiac massage and prolonged artificial respiration. N Engl J Med 264:36–38
Rindfleisch E (1862) Ein Fall von Blitzschlag. Arch Path Anat Physiol Klin Med 25:417–419
Schaidt G (1977) Spuren an Kleidungsstücken beim Blitzunfall. Arch Kriminol 159:93–96
Schniers E (2005) Schädigungen und Tod nach Blitzschlag – eine Synopsis aus rechtsmedizinischer Sicht. Universität Rostock, Rostock, Med Diss
Sellier K (1975) Schäden und Tod durch Elektrizität. In: Mueller B (Eds) Gerichtliche Medizin, 2nd edn. Teil 1. Springer, Berlin Heidelberg New York, pp 538–563
Stricker W (1861) Die Wirkung des Blitzes auf den menschlichen Körper. Arch Path Anat Physiol Klin Med 20:45–79
Stricker W (1863) Neue Untersuchungen und Beobachtungen über die Wirkung des Blitzes auf den menschlichen Körper. Arch Path Anat Physiol Klin Med 28:552–555
Stricker W (1872) Der Blitz und seine Wirkungen. Lüderitz'sche Verlagsbuchhandlung, Berlin
Uman MA (1986) All about lightning. Dover Publications, New York
Weimann W, Prokop O (1963) Atlas der gerichtlichen Medizin. Volk und Gesundheit, Berlin
Wetli CW (1996) Keraunopathology. An analysis of 45 fatalities. Am J Forensic Med Pathol 17:89–98
Zack F, Büttner A (2020a) Blitzunfall Teil 1: Physikalische und epidemiologische Aspekte, Energieübertragung und Schädigungen nach überlebten Ereignissen. Rechtsmedizin 30:267–278
Zack F, Büttner A (2020b) Blitzunfall Teil 2: Pathophysiologische und diagnostische Aspekte bei tödlichen Ereignissen. Rechtsmedizin 30:345–353
Zack F, Hammer U, Klett I, Wegener R (1997) Myocardial injury due to lightning. Int J Legal Med 110:326–328
Zack F, Rammelsberg JO, Graf B, Büttner A (2010) Tod durch Blitzschlag – und wieder unter einem Baum. Rechtsmedizin 20:108–110
Zack F, Raphael T, Kupfer J, Jokuszies A, Vogt PM, Büttner A, Püschel K, Schalke B, Todt M, Dettmeyer R (2013) Vier Todesopfer nach einem Blitzunfall auf einem Golfplatz. Rechtsmedizin 23:114–118

3 Meteorological and Electrical Engineering Basics

3.1 Thunderstorms

Thunderstorms are widespread weather phenomena, in which there are electrical discharges in the form of lightning and sound waves in the form of thunder. They often involve heavy precipitation and gusty winds, which can also reach storm strength. Thunderstorms occur when warm moist air masses rise to great heights and there is a temperature difference between the stationary and the rising air (Heidler and Stimper 2009). There are constantly and simultaneously about 2000 thunderstorms on Earth (Rakov and Uman 2006).

In meteorology, the four types of thunderstorms cold front thunderstorms, heat thunderstorms, orographic thunderstorms, and warm front thunderstorms are distinguished from each other.

For Europe, the time-of-day independent *cold front thunderstorms,* which can occur throughout the year, are the most common type of thunderstorm. In this case, large cold air masses push under the existing warm air and push it upwards. This results in extensive thunderstorm fronts and considerable train speeds, so that relatively large areas are affected by these thunderstorms.

The second most common type of thunderstorm in Germany and numerous European countries are the *heat thunderstorms*. They are caused by intensive solar radiation of the earth's surface and the near-surface air layers and occur most frequently in the afternoon or in the evening hours of a summer day.

Orographic thunderstorms can occur regardless of the season in the transition regions from the lowlands to the mountains. The ascent of the warm moist air is caused by the wind stream against the mountain.

F. Zack, *Accidents Caused by Lightning Strikes*,
https://doi.org/10.1007/978-3-662-71066-1_3

Warm front thunderstorms are rare and are caused by a sliding of warm air masses onto existing cold air. In Europe, warm front thunderstorms occur preferably in winter, when warm moist sea air meets continental cold air.

The tropics have the highest frequency of thunderstorms with 100–200 days per year and location. From here, the frequency of thunderstorms decreases with increasing latitudes towards the poles. This tendency is also found in Germany. While in the south of Germany about 20–35 thunderstorm days per year and location are recorded, in northern Germany it is about half as many.

In Central Europe, the most thunderstorm days per month are found in the warm season, especially in the months of May to August. The thunderstorms occur most frequently in the afternoon and evening hours (Heidler and Stimper 2009).

3.2 Lightning

Lightning is caused by the separation of electric charge carriers in thunderclouds (Cumulonimbus, Fig. 8.1). In this process, voltages of several tens of millions of volts can occur between different clouds or between a cloud and the earth (Hasse et al. 2006). When a discharge occurs, electric currents of up to 200,000 A flow. This results in a sudden heating of the air by the lightning current, leading to an explosion of the lightning channel (Heidler and Stimper 2009). Not infrequently, an extremely short but intense charge exchange is followed by further discharges in the same lightning channel as subsequent lightning with current strengths of several thousand amperes (Heidler and Stimper 2009). Furthermore, so-called long-term currents with comparatively lower current strengths of a few hundred amperes, but longer duration of up to 500 ms, also occur. These transport large amounts of charge and are therefore of high relevance for fires and health damage to humans. The hot plasma core of the lightning channel, which has a diameter of a few millimeters to a few centimeters, can reach temperatures of over 30,000 °C (Heidler and Cvetic 2002; Rakov and Uman 2006).

There are cloud-to-ground lightning, cloud-to-cloud lightning, cloud-to-air lightning and lightning within a cloud (Fig. 3.1). Apart from aviation and space travel, only cloud-to-ground lightning is dangerous for human life and health. In particular, space research has revealed that there are various forms of discharge above thunderclouds (Heidler and Stimper 2009; Rakov 2021).

In terms of charges, positive and negative cloud-to-ground lightning are distinguished, with negatively charged lightning being the most common and having technical parameters that exceed human imagination.

A typical small thunderstorm system generates a lightning strike to the ground every 20–30 s for 40–60 min and covers an area of typically about 100–300 km^2. This corresponds approximately to a circle on the ground with a radius between 6 and 10 km.

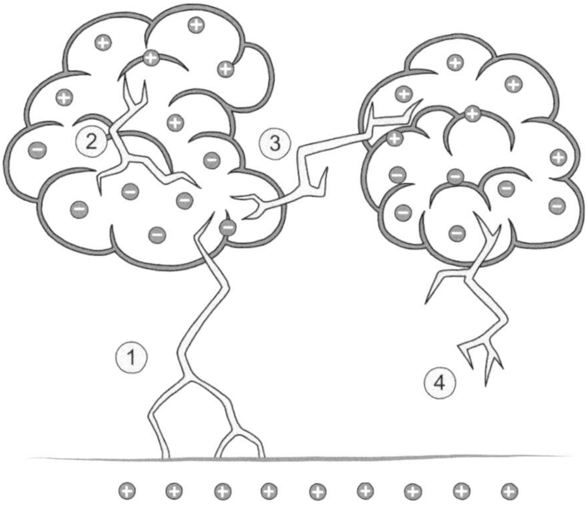

Fig. 3.1 The different types of lightning are cloud-to-ground lightning (1), lightning within a cloud (2), cloud-to-cloud lightning (3), and cloud-to-air lightning (4). (Own illustration)

Large storm systems can generate more than one ground lightning per second over areas that are 100 times larger (Uman 2008).

Lightning can harm a person in rain or snowfall, but also in the precipitation-free area under a cloudless sky. The latter lightning strikes are called "bolt from the blue phenomenon" and are caused by a non-vertical discharge of the electrical discharge from the thunderstorm cell (Blumenthal 2022; Cherington et al. 1997; Kleiter et al. 2007). In the technical literature, there is a documented accident that occurred at a distance of 16 km from the nearest registered thunderstorm cell (Cherington et al. 1997). About 10% of cloud-to-ground lightning strikes reach the ground in a precipitation-free area (Walsh et al. 2013; Uman 1986). However, most cloud-to-ground lightning strikes have a length of about 3–4 km (Uman 1986).

3.3 Lightning Detection Systems

With the help of lightning detection systems, the timing, impact location, and intensity of lightning can be recorded. The registered data primarily serve scientific and economic interests, e.g., in the fields or sectors of meteorology, air traffic, energy supply, telecommunications, and insurance. But also for doctors, other natural scientists, investigators, and other interested parties, lightning detection systems are a relevant support in diagnosing or reconstructing an accident.

Lightning detection systems are divided into the categories local, regional, and global, which differ in their ranges:

a) **Local Lightning Detection Systems**

The range of local lightning detection systems is a maximum of 100 km. Since there is direct visual contact between the sensors and the lightning channel, the range is limited solely by the curvature of the earth.

b) **Regional Lightning Detection Systems**

The range of regional lightning detection systems is up to about 1000 km. The lightning detection systems consist of at least six measuring stations and a central station that evaluates and stores the transmitted measurement data.

This system form has the greatest practical relevance, as the possible range often covers the area of an entire country. The regional lightning detection systems are called, for example, BLIDS for Germany, ALDIS for Austria, and MeteoSwitzerland for Switzerland. To improve the performance of regional lightning detection systems, 32 European countries have now joined together in the "European Cooperation for Lightning Detection" (EUCLID) founded in 2001 (see Chap. 7). But also numerous other countries of the world, some of which also cooperate with each other, have regional lightning detection systems (Guha et al. 2021).

c) **Global Lightning Detection Systems**

The range of global lightning detection systems is several thousand km. In this type of detection systems, the regional systems are supported by satellites. The global lightning detection systems provide an overview of the supra-regional thunderstorm activity and the direction of the storm fronts. They primarily serve meteorology and climate research (Heidler and Stimper 2009).

References

Blumenthal R (2022) Lightning metallization injury. Am J Forensic Med Pathol 43:e93–e95

Cherington M, Krider EP, Yarnell PR, Breed DW (1997) A bolt from the blue: lightning strike to the head. Neurology 48:683–686

Guha A, Liu Y, Williams E, Schumann C, Hunt H (2021) Lightning, detection and warning. In: Gomes C (Eds) Lightning. Science, engineering, and economic implications for developing countries. Springer, Singapore, pp 37–77

Hasse P, Wiesinger J, Zischank W (2006) Handbuch für Blitzschutz und Erdung, 5th edn. Pflaum, München

Heidler F, Cvetic J (2002) A class of analytical functions to study the lightning effects associated with the current front. ETEP 12:141–150

Heidler F, Stimper K (2009) Blitz und Blitzschutz. VDE, Berlin Offenbach

Kleiter I, Luerding R, Dienhofer G, Rek H, Bogdahn U, Schalke B (2007) A lightning strike to the head causing a visual cortex defect with simple and complex visual hallucinations. J Neurol Neurosurg Psychiatry 78:423–426

Rakov VA (2021) Lightning, the science. In: Gomes C (Ed) Lightning. Science, engineering, and economic implications for developing countries. Springer, Singapore, pp 1–36

Rakov VA, Uman MA (2006) Lightning. Physics and effects. Cambridge University Press, Cambridge New York Melbourne Madrid Cape Town Singapore Sao Paulo

Uman MA (1986) All about lightning. Dover Publication, New York

Uman MA (2008) The art and science of lightning protection. Cambridge University Press, Cambridge New York Melbourne Madrid Cape Town Singapore Sao Paulo Delhi

Walsh KM, Cooper MA, Holle R, Rakov VA, Roeder WP, Ryan M (2013) National athletic trainers' association safety for athletics and recreation. J Athl Train 48:258–270

4 Mechanisms of Energy Transfer

Lightning accidents are characterized, in contrast to accidents with technical high voltage, by an extremely high current strength and a very short exposure duration. Injuries result from the impact of electrical energy, high temperatures, mechanical energy in the form of the explosive expansion of air after heating, or the bright light (Blumenthal 2021; Pollak and Thierauf 2015; Rakov and Uman 2006; Uman 1986, 1992; Zack et al. 2007). The energy of the lightning can be transferred to a person or groups of people in various ways and can also lead to injuries in the form of a magnetic field. Numerous accidents involve a combination of different mechanisms (Blumenthal et al. 2012; Cherington et al. 1998; Cooper 2000; Pollak and Thierauf 2015; Ritenour et al. 2008; Association of Electrical Engineering Electronics Information Technology 2012; Zack et al. 2007; Zack and Büttner 2020a). The individual mechanisms of energy transfer to humans are presented below (Table 4.1).

> **Note** Human lightning strike injuries can result from the impact of electrical, mechanical and/or thermal energy as well as from bright light.

4.1 Direct Strike

In the case of a direct strike ("direct strike", "direct hit"), which has the greatest potential for human danger, the main part of the current passes through the body. Lightning entry points are often found on the head and occasionally lightning exit marks in the form of hole-like electrical discharges on the feet (Fig. 4.1). The lethality of such accidents is relatively high (Blumenthal et al. 2012; Cooper 2000; Pollak and Thierauf 2015; Ritenour et al. 2008; Association of Electrical Engineering Electronics Information Technology 2012; Whitcomb 2002; Zack et al. 2007, 2016).

F. Zack, *Accidents Caused by Lightning Strikes*,
https://doi.org/10.1007/978-3-662-71066-1_4

Table 4.1 Mechanisms of possible energy transfers in a lightning strike accident. (Own representation)

Mechanism	Brief description
Direct hit	Current flow through the body
Contact voltage	Lightning strike into an object being touched by the victim
Side flash	Lightning strike into an object, e.g., tree, with "jumping" of the energy
Step voltage	Damage due to an obtained step voltage near the lightning strike
Conductor-mediated lightning accident	Current flow to the victim via electrical lines, touch is not a prerequisite
Upward lightning	Damage due to current flow from the ground towards the sky
Barotrauma	Damage due to explosive shock/pressure wave
Blinding	Damage due to the bright light of the lightning channel
Secondary accident mechanism	Damage due to lightning-induced fire, falling branches or similar

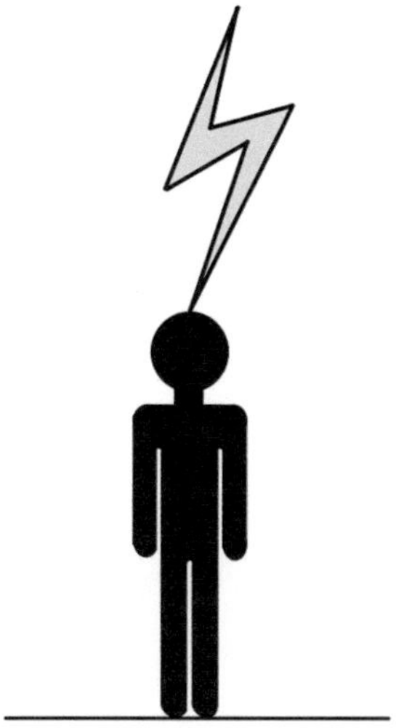

Fig. 4.1 In a direct strike, the impact site is often in the head-neck area and the exit site in the foot area. The electric current flows through the body in this case. (Own illustration)

Case Study

A 13-year-old boy received a direct strike to the left side of his neck on a school playground in England, with exit burns on both feet. An apparently uninjured friend observed how the victim fell to the ground and remained motionless. When he touched him, he felt hot. A school staff member assessed the situation and began immediate cardiopulmonary resuscitation on the unresponsive boy. Alerted paramedics transported the victim to the emergency room of a clinic, continuing resuscitation treatment throughout, which was reached 18 minutes after the lightning strike.

Findings on the day of admission: Glasgow Coma Scale 3, sinus tachycardia (140 beats/min), left tympanic membrane rupture, weak breathing, cold extremities, respiratory and metabolic acidosis (pH 6.9), increase in serum creatine kinase (CK) to a maximum of 1164 IU/L (reference range: 0–120 IU/L), no pathological findings in echocardiography and electrocardiogram (ECG), superficial burns of the neck, chest region and abdomen on the left side, superficial burns on the left foot and deep burns on the right foot, open wound on the chin from falling, tears in the jacket and trousers on the left side and the left shoe.

Therapy and clinical course in the intensive care unit: intubation, mechanical ventilation, volume substitution, forced diuresis, treatment of skin burns with dry gauze dressings, surgical suturing of the chin wound, on the 3rd day extubation and normalization of CK. On the 4th day, transfer to a regular ward due to existing dysphasia and muscle weakness on the right side. No further course was reported (Courtman et al. 2003). ◀

4.2 Side Flash

A side flash or side splash occurs when the lightning first strikes another object, e.g. a tree, and part of the energy is transferred to a person nearby (Fig. 4.2). The lethality of a side flash is also considered relatively high (Ritenour et al. 2008; Whitcomb 2002; Zack et al. 1997, 2016).

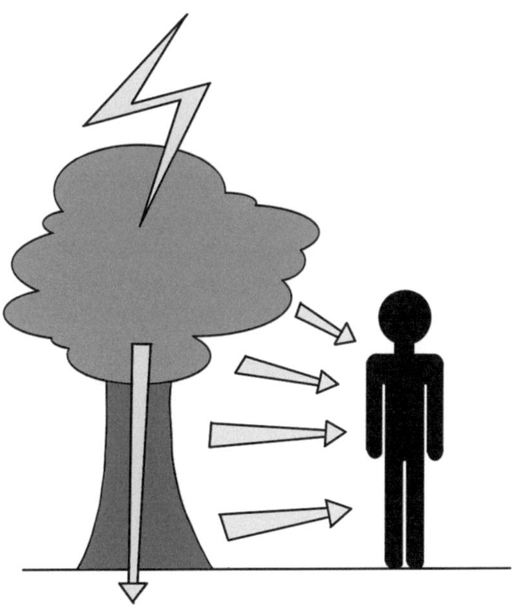

Fig. 4.2 In a side flash, the lightning strikes another object, in most cases a tree, and part of the energy is transferred to the victim nearby. (Own illustration)

Case Study

On a day in May 1995, numerous participants of a sports festival in Rastow, Mecklenburg-Vorpommern (Germany), were surprised by a thunderstorm with heavy rain. Most of the people involved ran into a supply tent set up next to the sports field. Lightning then struck a poplar, which was part of a row of trees on the edge of the sports field, leaving a vertical burn mark on the tree bark down to the grass. In the tent, which was 1.50 m away from the struck tree, a 27-year-old man was seriously injured. After immediate loss of consciousness and ventricular fibrillation, he was successfully resuscitated, intubated, artificially ventilated and taken to a hospital, where he died 5 days after the accident due to irreversible hypoxic brain damage. The autopsy showed no damage to the skin or body hair of the victim. After the soft tissues were prepared, the left pectoral muscle and the heart showed extensive thermal damage in the form of coagulations. The tree had taken the direct hit, but the victim was too close to the tree and the air resistance and the tent sheet were not suitable to protect the man from the high energy in the vicinity of the direct hit. It was the first case of damage caused by a side flash described in the German technical literature (Zack et al. 1997). ◀

4.3 Step Voltage

In an accident caused by step voltage (also known as "ground strike", "stride potential", "grounding", "ground current effect", "ground current electrocution"), the affected person is located up to 50 m away from the lightning strike site with their legs on the ground. The lightning channel discharges its electrical voltage into the ground at the point of impact. This creates a so-called voltage funnel, where the voltage continuously decreases with increasing distance from the lightning strike. A potential difference arises between both feet, especially at a considerable distance. The current enters the body through one foot and exits through the other (Fig. 4.3). Health damage caused by step voltage is usually survived in humans because the current does not pass through the heart. However, in larger mammals, step voltage can lead to death due to the greater distances between the legs (Cooper 2000; Panse 1925; Rakov and Uman 2006; Ritenour et al. 2008; Sellier 1975; VDE 2012; Whitcomb et al. 2002; Zack et al. 2007, 2016).

No case report could be found in the medical literature in which a human victim, unlike large mammals, had demonstrably died solely from step voltage (Blumenthal 2021; Cooper et al. 2017; Zack and Büttner 2020b).

Of the 10 deaths from step voltage reported in a non-medical study from Germany, not a single deceased person was autopsied or postmortem examined by an expert. The assess-

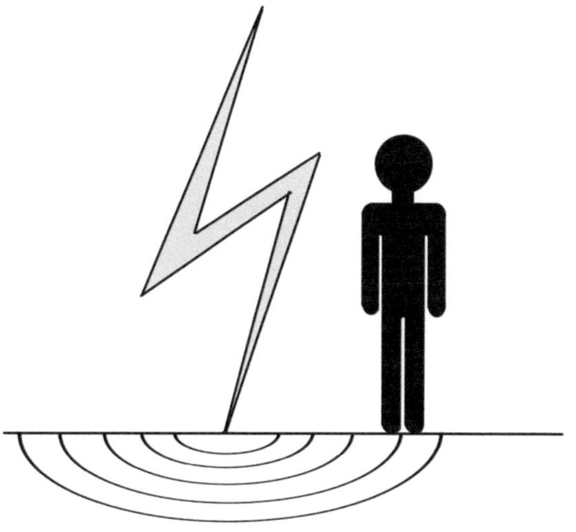

Fig. 4.3 In the case of step voltage, the victim is walking or standing in the immediate vicinity of a lightning strike to the ground. (Own illustration)

ment was preliminary and based on statements from witnesses, some of whom had been injured themselves, and must be retrospectively doubted (Bremer 2024; Harms 1956).

Lichtenberg et al. (1993) reported on 12 patients who had suffered an injury from step voltage. All victims showed paresthesia of the lower extremities with numbness, burning, tingling and/or muscle weakness. No patient had ST elevation or QTc prolongation in a derived ECG. In 3 of the 12 victims, the ECG showed nonspecific ST-T wave changes. The disease courses were uncomplicated and the cardiological follow-up examinations revealed no abnormalities.

Many victims of a lightning accident caused by step voltage do not even need to be hospitalized, as the symptoms and complaints often regress in a short time (Diehl 2008; Dollinger 1985; Duppel et al. 2009; Zack et al. 1997, 2009).

Case Example

After an accident caused by a lightning strike into a group of trees at a public swimming pool in Baden-Württemberg (Germany), a 35-year-old man was slightly confused at the scene. He had a stable circulation and complained of numbness in both legs. The thigh and foot pulses were not palpable. Furthermore, there was symmetrical motor weakness and dysesthesias on palpation in the left lumbar and sacral area. This was followed by a rapid regression of symptoms within the first 2 hours after the accident, except for the dysesthesias. The further course was uncomplicated. Two years after the accident, the victim still suffered from occasional pain in both legs (Graber et al. 1996). ◀

4.4 Contact Voltage

A contact voltage ("contact injury") is present when lightning strikes an object that is in direct contact with a lightning victim. The current then flows through a victim if this person represents the path of least resistance (Fig. 4.4). In individual cases, fatal accidents have also been reported (Cooper 2000; Ritenour et al. 2008; VDE 2020, Whitcomb et al. 2002; Zack et al. 2007, 2016).

Case Study

At the moment a 24-year-old truck driver in Minnesota (USA) was coupling a trailer to a tractor unit, lightning struck the truck. The man was thrown several meters away but remained conscious. He suffered a burn to his left hand and was disoriented afterwards, so he was taken to the emergency room of a clinic. There he showed a permanent sinus tachycardia. No further pathological findings were detected in the victim.

After 1.5 months, the victim of the lightning accident developed palpitations, episodic pain in the upper extremities (lasting 5-10 seconds), increased diaphoresis, and arterial hypertension (at least 160/115 mmHg).

After 3 months, a post-traumatic stress disorder occurred in the form of anxiety, insomnia, general restlessness, fine motor and memory disorders, and headaches. Traditional physiotherapy and occupational therapy did not improve the symptoms. As a result, a change in therapy management was initiated 4.5 months after the accident, with the start of psychotherapy, functional rehabilitation treatment, and administration of clonidine. As a result, there was a significant improvement in symptoms (Parsaik et al. 2013). ◀

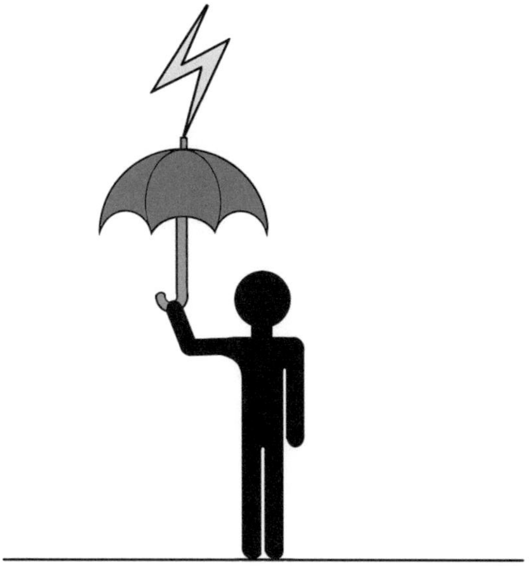

Fig. 4.4 In a contact effect, the victim touches an object, e.g., an umbrella, which is struck by lightning. (Own illustration)

4.5 Wire-Mediated Lightning Accident

In a wire-mediated lightning accident ("wire mediated lightning injury"), a person can be injured or killed after the electrical energy of a lightning strike has entered a telephone or electrical line and the accident victim is using a corded telephone or devices with a cord connection to the electrical grid. Direct contact with the power line is not a prerequisite for damage (Fig. 4.5) (Blanco-Pampin et al. 1997; Dinakaran et al. 1998; Pollak and Thierauf 2015; Zack and Büttner 2020a).

Case Study

In the early morning hours of a day in July 1995, a 55-year-old man was found dead in his bed in Spain. The coroner initially suspected a natural death. The isolated house had been struck by lightning two years earlier. At around 4 a.m. the previous night, there had been a thunderstorm in this region again. With this knowledge, a second post-mortem examination of the deceased was carried out, this time by forensic doctors. They found that the mast of the television antenna on the property, which was about 8 m high and towered over the roof of the single-story country house, had been struck by lightning. The electrical energy of the lightning had then entered the house via cable lines and destroyed or damaged the television, a water heater, and numerous electrical lines. In the bedroom of the house, the lightning struck a surface-mounted

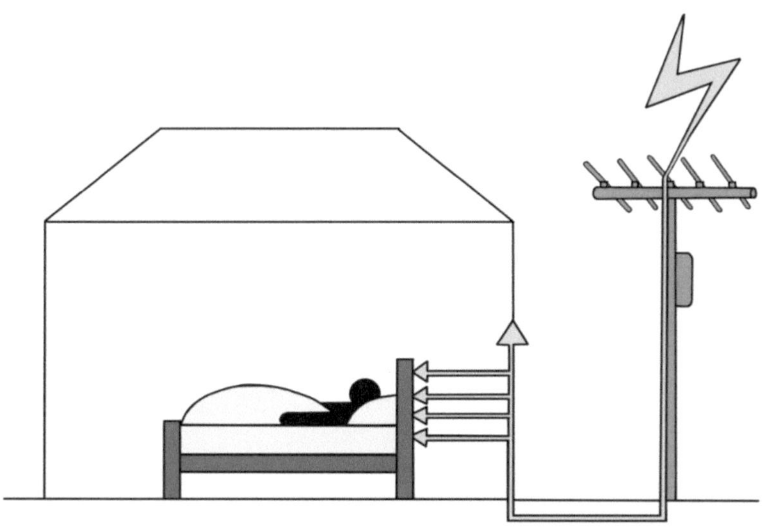

Fig. 4.5 In a wire-mediated lightning accident, a person can be harmed by a lightning strike that has entered the electrical installations of a house, even without touching the electrical line. (Own illustration)

line about 10 cm from the head of the wooden bed in which the man had died. The investigators found thermal damage to the headboard of the bed frame, which was made of 2 cm thick wood, as well as burns on the pillow, sheets, and mattress. The skin of the deceased man showed superficial injuries on the right shoulder and Lichtenberg figures on the upper body. These findings led the forensic doctors to the correct diagnosis of "death by lightning strike".

The energy of the lightning reached the victim of the case study via the antenna and the surface-mounted electrical lines, without the man touching a line with his body. Therefore, the contact voltage (contact effect) as a type of energy transfer is not considered for this tragic accident, so the wire-mediated energy transfer should be considered as an independent mechanism of damage to a person and was included in the enumeration (Blanco-Pampin et al. 1997; Zack et al. 2007). ◀

4.6 Upward Lightning

In the case of an upward lightning or a leader discharge ("upward streamer"), a victim of an accident is injured by oppositely directed charges that run from the earth's surface or from the head of the accident victim towards the cloud (Fig. 4.6). This form of energy transfer has only been described once in the medical literature. The accident victim died at the scene of the event (Cooper 2002).

Case Study

On a day in September 1998, a four-person team in North Carolina (USA) was working on expanding a power station. The men were working at a road junction under trees. When it began to thunder, the shift supervisor, against the will of the other

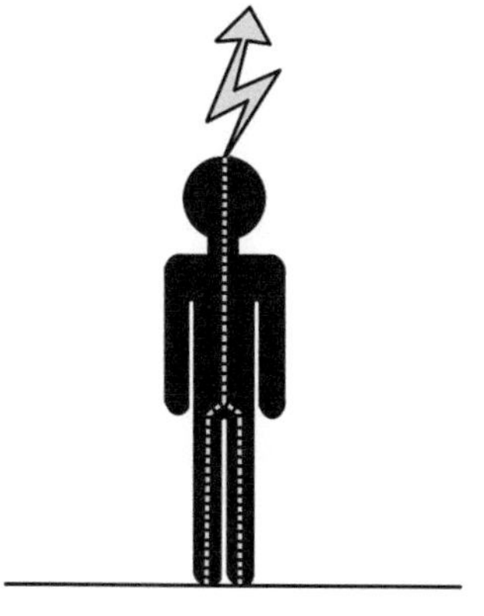

Fig. 4.6 In the case of an upward lightning ("upward streamer"), a person can be injured or killed by electrical charges that are directed from the earth's surface or from the head of the victim towards the cloud. (Own illustration)

three men, ordered the work to continue. The person in charge himself was kneeling between a transformer box and a telephone installation column when an employee felt a tingling sensation in his left side of the body. While there was a loud bang, another employee observed a whitish flash in the area of the head and right shoulder of the shift supervisor. He then said that he was not feeling well and collapsed. Two employees immediately began resuscitation. Whether cardiac massage was also started immediately is not mentioned in the report. The paramedics who arrived 7 minutes later found a ventricular fibrillation of the heart and continued the resuscitation measures, but without success (Cooper 2002). ◀

4.7 Barotrauma

Regardless of the electrical charge, a victim of a lightning-related accident can also suffer health damage from other forms of energy. In this context, a barotrauma often occurs (Fig. 4.7) (Angerer et al. 2009; Blumenthal 2021; VDE 2012).

A detailed examination of the mechanisms of a lightning-related barotrauma does not yet exist in the medical literature. A subsequent inquiry to the head of the Lightning and Overvoltage Protection department at the Technical University of Ilmenau, Germany, provided the following explanation, which is also understandable from a medical point of view, for the frequently observed eardrum ruptures and tearing of worn clothing in accident victims.

The barotrauma is caused by the sudden heating of the air, which causes a shock/pressure wave around the plasma channel of the lightning. This wave then becomes an intense sound wave at some distance, which can be heard as thunder at an even greater

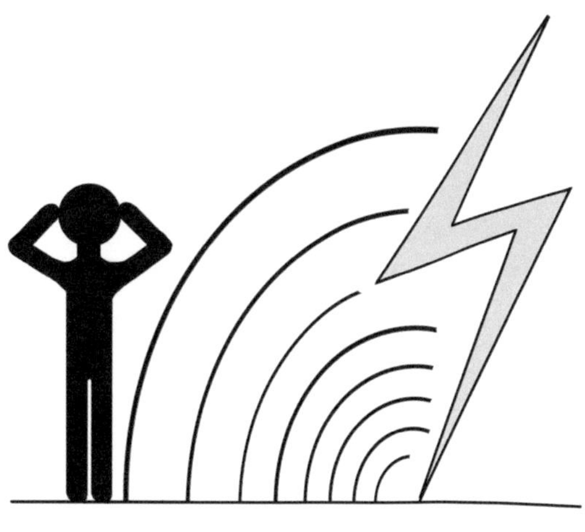

Fig. 4.7 In a barotrauma, a person can be thrown through the air and/or injured at the hearing organ by the shock/pressure wave, which is due to a sudden heating of the air in the plasma channel. (Own illustration)

distance. This shock and pressure wave spreads in all directions around the lightning channel. When the wave hits a nearby person, they can be knocked over or even thrown away by the high surface pressure, without necessarily tearing their clothing.

The situation is different when a person is injured either by a direct hit or a side flash. In this case, the plasma/slide discharge occurs either on the skin, between skin and clothing, or on the clothing due to the high resistance of the human body. The plasma/slide discharge corresponds to the continuation of the lightning channel directly on the surface of a person. Here too, there is a sudden heating of the air around the lightning channel and the formation of a shock/pressure wave. In this process, the victim's eardrums are often injured and the victim's worn clothing is almost always torn. The damage can occur both when the lightning runs between skin and clothing, and in cases of slide discharge on the outside of the clothing. In the first case, the shock/pressure wave moving away from the lightning channel causes the tears. In the case of discharge on the outside of the clothing, the outward pressure pulse into the air behind it, on the clothing, causes a strong negative pressure or suction ("suction force"). If moisture is also present due to rain or sweat, which is likely in a heat thunderstorm, the aforementioned effects are further intensified. The liquid water of the moisture is suddenly vaporized by the extreme heating, i.e., converted into the gaseous state, which corresponds to a significant volume increase. This makes the amplitude and the mechanical effect larger. This is probably why noticeable tears can be observed even with relatively low-energy lightning if moisture is present. Whether damage occurs or not also depends on the material of the clothing. In particular, the anatomical and physiological properties of the skin are likely to be responsible for the fact that it does not show similar tears in relation to human clothing (M. Rock, personal communication, January 12, 2023).

Case Example

During a car journey in Bavaria (Germany) in 2007, a 44-year-old driver's car was struck by lightning. The car, which protected the driver from damage by the electrical energy as a Faraday cage, subsequently showed a failure of the entire vehicle electronics, paint damage on the roof, and thermal damage to the wheel covers. The driver suffered a severe acoustic trauma (barotrauma) with bilateral otalgia, tinnitus, and hearing loss on the right side. After infusion therapy, the inner ear hearing loss improved after 2 weeks, while the tinnitus persisted for more than 6 months (Angerer et al. 2009). ◀

4.8 Blinding

Through the blinding of the bright light from the lightning channel, the eyes of a victim can be damaged (Kleiter et al. 2007; Mason and Crocett 2000).

Case Study

On her way home from school, a 14-year-old girl in Canada saw a bright light and found herself sitting on the ground the next moment. She appeared in the emergency room of a clinic with pain in her eyes, left shoulder, and both legs. She also complained of abnormal sensations (numbness, tingling) in her legs.

Examination findings: Decreased strength (4/5) and sensory disturbances of the right lower leg, limping gait, in the EKG atrioventricular block (AV block) of the 1st degree.

Monitoring. An ophthalmological consultation yielded an unremarkable examination result.

Discharge after 2 days with persistence of bright light appearances in both eyes, paresthesias in the lower extremities, and a 1st degree AV block. Discharge medication: Amitriptyline (Mason and Crocett 2000). ◄

4.9 Secondary Accident Mechanism

Furthermore, individuals can be secondarily injured by different consequences of a lightning strike. Injuries or death can be caused, for example, by a fire caused by the extreme temperatures of the lightning channel (Fig. 4.8) or by splintered parts of a struck tree (Blumenthal 2021; Bremer 2024; Harms 1956; Holle 2010; Holle et al. 2005; Ritenour et al. 2008).

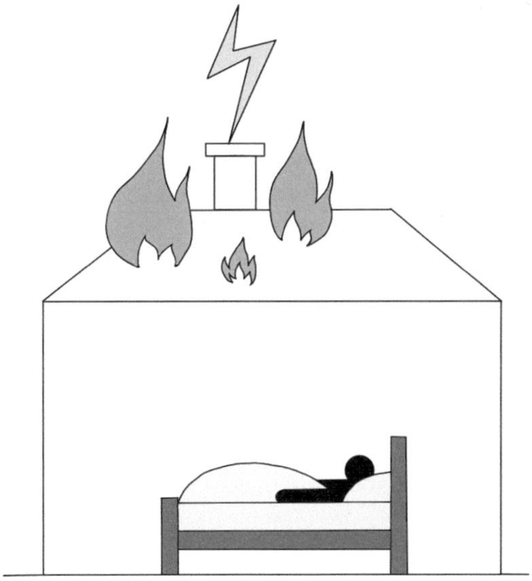

Fig. 4.8 A lightning strike can also secondarily harm the health of individuals, e.g., by triggering a fire. (Own illustration)

Case Study

On a morning in August 1955, an accident with secondary damage occurred at a lake in Schleswig-Holstein (Germany). Six people were sitting under the awning of a tent during a thunderstorm when lightning struck a poplar tree about 4 m away and nearly 30 m high. The tree was part of a row of poplars and had a trunk diameter of about 1 m. The lightning shattered the trunk, causing trunk parts and branches to fall to the ground within a radius of 15 m. A 35-year-old man was hit on the head by a splintered piece of tree about 1.50 m long and weighing 8 kg while sitting and died at the scene of the accident. The coroner diagnosed a severe traumatic brain injury as the cause of death due to bleeding from the mouth, nose, and ears. Of the other 5 people, 4 had health impairments such as confusion, paralysis, an arm fracture, and pain and were treated in a hospital (Bremer 2024). ◀

4.10 Magnetic Field

Furthermore, there is the hypothesis that the magnetic field occurring during a lightning strike can cause electrical currents resulting in asystole or ventricular fibrillation in the victim. This is particularly supposed to apply to severely injured individuals who do not show any characteristic findings from the lightning strike externally after the accident (Cherington et al. 1998; Wetli 1996).

Case Study

Four golfers were under a tree during a thunderstorm in the USA when lightning struck the tree. Two men were briefly unconscious, one player complained of burns at the spots where he carried clubs and other metal objects, and a 32-year-old man suffered a cardiac arrest. A doctor who was nearby immediately began cardiopulmonary resuscitation measures. The man was taken to a clinic but remained comatose and died 18 days later due to hypoxic brain damage. Since he showed no external injuries from electrical current flow, Cherington et al. (1998) hypothesized that a person can also be so severely damaged by the magnetic field existing in the vicinity of a cloud-to-ground lightning strike that a cardiac arrest occurs. ◀

A single form of energy transfer or a combination of different mechanisms can be responsible for a lightning accident causing health damage to a person (Johnstone et al. 1986; Zack et al. 1997).

In the evaluation of accidents caused by lightning strikes with health damage to individuals published in the technical literature, there is often no indication of the determined or assumed energy transfer path. Possibly for the reasons mentioned, there are no reliable

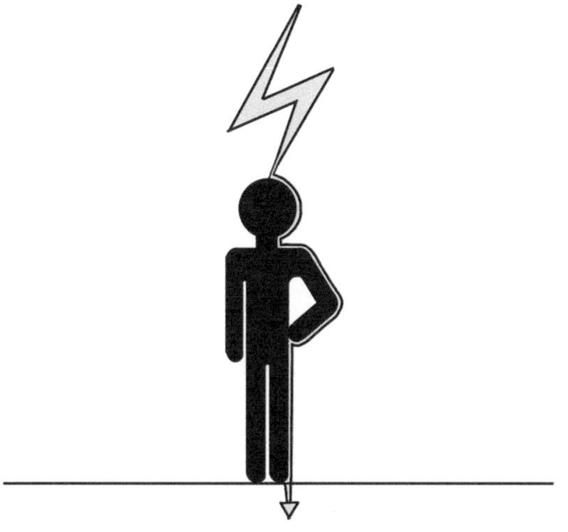

Fig. 4.9 In a surface effect ("skin effect", "flashover phenomenon"), the main part of the electrical lightning current is discharged into the ground along the body surface in the form of a sliding discharge. (Own illustration)

statistics in the technical literature about accidents with personal injuries about the frequencies of the occurrence of the different energy transfer mechanisms.

In the case of a surface effect ("skin effect", "flashover phenomenon"), it is assumed that the main part of the electrical energy of the lightning channel is discharged into the ground along the body surface in the form of a sliding discharge. The causes are considered to be the drop in electrical voltage due to skin resistance and the extremely short exposure time. The skin effect is a significant reason why lightning strikes can be survived. However, it is not an independent energy transfer mechanism (Fig. 4.9) (Reimann and Prokop 1980; Weimann and Prokop 1963; Zack et al. 2007). The surface effect is supposed to occur preferentially in soaked individuals (Blumenthal 2021).

▶ **Note** In an accident caused by a lightning strike, the electrical energy can harm a person through various mechanisms. Accidents are described by a direct hit, a side flash, a contact voltage, a step voltage, a wire-mediated energy transfer, or an upward lightning. The different forms can also occur in combination. Furthermore, people can also suffer health damage in such events due to thermal and/or mechanical energy as well as blinding of the bright light.

References

Angerer F, Hoppe U, Schick B (2009) Blitzeinschlag in einen PKW mit Schädigung des Hörorgans. HNO 57:1081–1084

Blanco-Pampin JM, Suarez-Penaranda JM, Rico-Boquete R, Concheira-Carro L (1997) An unusual case of death by lightning. J Forensic Sci 42:942–944

Blumenthal R (2021) Injuries and deaths from lightning. J Clin Pathol 74:279–284

Blumenthal R, Jandrell IR, West NJ (2012) Does a sixth mechanism exist to explain lightning injuries? Investigating a possible new injury mechanism to determine the cause of injuries related to close lightning flashes. Am J Forensic Med Pathol 33:222–226

Bremer L (2024) Retrospektive Analyse einer historischen Fallsammlung von letalen Unfällen durch Blitzschlag in der Bundesrepublik Deutschland im Zeitraum 1951–1965 aus rechtsmedizinischer Sicht. Universität Rostock, Rostock im Druck, Med Diss

Cherington M, Wachtel H, Yarnell PR (1998) Could lightning injury be magnetically induced? Lancet 351:1788

Cooper MA (2002) A fifth mechanism of lightning injury. Acad Emerg Med 9:172–174

Cooper MA, Andrews CJ, Holle RL, Blumenthal R, Navarette-Aldana N (2017) Lightning-related injuries and safety. In: Auerbach P, Cushing T, Harris N (eds) Auerbach's wilderness medicine. 7th edn. Elsevier, Philadelphia, pp 71–117

Courtman SP, Wilson PM, Mok Q (2003) Case report of a 13-year-old struck by lightning. Paediatr Anaesth 13:76–79

Diehl J (2008) Eine Meldung und ihre Geschichte—warum ein Blitz 19 Fußballtrainer gleichzeitig traf. Spiegel 27:55

Dinakaran S, Desai SP, Elsom DM (1998) Telephone-mediated lightning injury causing cataract. Injury 29:645–646

Dollinger SJ (1985) Lightning-strike disaster among children. Br J Med Psychol 58:375–383

Duppel H, Löbermann M, Reisinger EC (2009) Aus heiterem Himmel vom Blitz getroffen. Dtsch Med Wochenschr 134:1214–1217

Graber J, Ummenhofer W, Herion H (1996) Lightning accident with eight victims: a case report and brief review of the literature. J Trauma 40:288–290

Harms W (1956) Personenblitzschäden. Elektromedizin 1:153–158

Holle RL (2010) Lightning-caused casualities in and near dwellings and other buildings. https://www.vaisala.com/sites/default/files/documents/9.Holle-Lightning-Caused.pdf. Accessed: 14 Dec 2022.

Holle RL, Lopez RE, Navarro BC (2005) Deaths, injuries, and damages from lightning in the United States in the 1890s in comparison with the 1990s. J Appl Meteorol 44:1563–1573

Johnstone BR, Harding DL, Hocking B (1986) Telephon-related lightning injury. Med J Aust 144:707–708

Kleiter I, Luerding R, Dienhofer G, Rek H, Bogdahn U, Schalke B (2007) A lightning strike to the head causing a visual cortex defect with simple and complex visual hallucinations. J Neurol Neurosurg Psychiatry 78:423–426

Lichtenberg R, Dries D, Ward K, Marshall W, Scanlon P (1993) Cardiovascular effects of lightning strikes. J Am Coll Cardiol 21:531–536

Mason AD, Crocett RK (2000) When lightning strikes … a case report and review of the literature. Int Pediatr 15:174–179

Panse F (1925) Über Schädigungen des Nervensystems durch Blitzschlag. Mschr Psychiat Neurol 59:323–338

Parsaik AK, Ahlskog JE, Singer W, Gelfman R, Sheldon SH, Seime RJ, Craft JM, Staab JP, Kantor B, Low PA (2013) Central hyperadrenergic state after lightning strike. Clin Auton Res 23:169–173

Pollak S, Thierauf A (2015) Elektrotraumen, Blitzschlag. In: Madea B (ed) Rechtsmedizin. 3rd edn. Springer, Berlin Heidelberg New York, pp 324–332

Rakov VA, Uman MA (2006) Lightning physics and effects. Cambridge University Press, Cambridge New York Melbourne Madrid Cape Town Singapore Sao Paulo

Reimann W, Prokop O (1980) Vademecum Gerichtsmedizin, 3rd edn. Volk und Gesundheit, Berlin

Ritenour AE, Morton MJ, McManus JG, Barillo DJ, Cancio LC (2008) Lightning injury: a review. Burns 34:585–594

Sellier K (1975) Schäden und Tod durch Elektrizität. In: Mueller B (ed) Gerichtliche Medizin, 2nd edn. Teil 1. Springer, Berlin Heidelberg New York, pp 538–563

Uman MA (1986) All about lightning. Dover Publications, New York

Uman MA (1992) Physics of lightning. In: Andrews CJ, Cooper MA, Darvenzia M, Mackerras D (eds) Lightning Injuries: electrical, medical, and legal aspects. CRC Press, Boca Raton Ann Arbor London Tokio, pp 5–21

Verband der Elektrotechnik Elektronik Informationstechnik e. V. (VDE) (2012) Unfälle durch Blitzeinwirkung. https://www.vde.com/resource/blob/936982/0f4076543f8f7ec91e3774536ca17ee0/merkblatt-blitzunfaelle-download-data.pdf. Accessed: 27 Jan 2020.

Weimann W, Prokop O (1963) Atlas der gerichtlichen Medizin. Volk und Gesundheit, Berlin

Wetli C (1996) Keraunopathology. An analysis of 45 fatalities. Am J Forensic Med Pathol 17:89–98

Whitcomb D, Martinez JA, Daberkow D (2002) Lightning injuries. South Med J 95:1331–1334

Zack F, Büttner A (2020a) Blitzunfall. Teil 1: Physikalische und epidemiologische Aspekte, Energieübertragung und Schädigungen nach überlebten Ereignissen. Rechtsmedizin 30:267–275

Zack F, Büttner A (2020b) Blitzunfall. Teil 2: Pathophysiologische und diagnostische Aspekte bei tödlichen Ereignissen. Rechtsmedizin 30:345–356

Zack F, Hammer U, Klett I, Wegener R (1997) Myocardial injury due to lightning. Int J Legal Med 110:326–328

Zack F, Rothschild MA, Wegener R (2007) Blitzunfall—Energieübertragungsmechanismen und medizinische Folgen. Dtsch Ärztebl 104:A3545–A3549

Zack F, Rummel J, Püschel K (2009) Blitzschläge auf Fußballplätzen. Eine unterschätzte Gefahr. Rechtsmedizin 19:77–82

Zack F, Puchstein S, Büttner A (2016) Letalität von Blitzunfällen. Rechtsmedizin 26:9–11

First Aid and Preclinical Emergency Medicine

5

As with almost every type of accident, first aid and preclinical emergency medicine at the accident site are of enormous relevance for the further clinical course and the consequences of lightning-related injuries. This type of accident has some peculiarities with regard to self-protection, triage, lay aid, and preclinical emergency medicine that need to be considered.

5.1 Self-Protection

Safety guidelines for thunderstorms have been published in various countries by interdisciplinary expert teams (Mackerras 1992; Association of Electrical Engineering Electronics Information Technology 2012; Zafren et al. 2005; Zimmermann et al. 2002). In contrast to an electrical accident at low or high voltage installations, there is no voltage immediately after a lightning strike at the event location. A continuous current flow through the victim or those rushing to provide first aid is thus excluded, unlike accidents in the field of technical electricity. Every victim of a lightning accident can be touched immediately without endangering one's own health through contact voltage (Hinkelbein et al. 2013; Association of Electrical Engineering Electronics Information Technology 2012).

Nevertheless, after a lightning accident with personal injury, self-protection is the primary concern for all first responders, especially in the case of ongoing lightning risk. This is particularly true for accidents that occur outdoors. The myth that lightning never strikes the same place twice, e.g., the location where first responders are operating, has long been debunked. For instance, the Empire State Building in New York City (USA) is struck by lightning an average of about 23 times per year. During a single storm,

F. Zack, *Accidents Caused by Lightning Strikes*,
https://doi.org/10.1007/978-3-662-71066-1_5

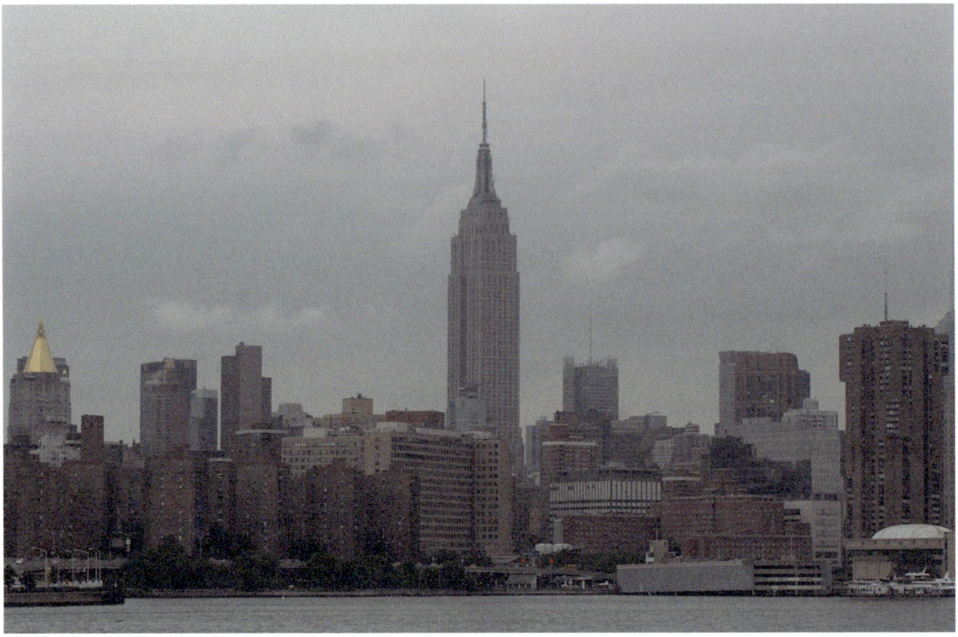

Fig. 5.1 The Empire State Building in New York City, including its antenna tip, which is 443 m tall, is struck by lightning several times a year. (Own illustration)

lightning struck the 443 m tall building, including the antenna tip, 8 times within 24 minutes (Uman 1986) (Fig. 5.1). There is no absolutely safe place for humans from lightning strike damage, but some places are safer than others (Holle et al. 1999; Rakov and Uman 2006). Ultimately, every first responder must minimize the risk of personal injury from a lightning strike. In the event of an accident with an injured person, this could be achieved, if possible, by approaching the victim closely and quickly transporting the person to an ambulance or a closed building. In the case of a mass casualty incident, the rescue teams will have to decide on the course of action situationally, depending on the circumstances on site, with absolute priority given to self-protection (Diepenseifen et al. 2009; Hinkelbein et al. 2013; Liebold et al. 2022; Association of Electrical Engineering Electronics Information Technology 2012). The helpers must decide at the scene of the accident whether immediate rescue of the affected persons is possible due to the number of injured persons, e.g., during a major event. Furthermore, it must be clarified whether immediate evacuation is even sensible in the face of potential self-endangerment of the rescue forces (Lederer and Kroesen 2005; Zafren et al. 2005; Zimmermann et al. 2002). If an evacuation as quickly as possible is carried out, all victims should be quickly brought to relatively safe places (see Chap. 8). The suitable environment for emergency medical treatment must be carefully selected. All places with an increased risk for humans to be struck by lightning should be avoided. These include wide open spaces, standalone trees, groups of trees or the edge of a forest, tall objects, proximity to high-voltage lines or other metal objects (exception: underneath bridges; see Chap. 8), waters, hills, mountains, and also tents. Thus, some potentially suitable places for the emergency medical treatment of numerous accident victims cannot be used (Holle et al. 1995; Leikin et al. 1997; Stütz et al. 2006; Zimmermann et al. 2002). In contrast, closed buildings with and without lightning protection systems, closed metal vehicles, and a rescue helicopter on the ground are suitable treatment locations in the event of a lightning risk (Zimmermann et al. 2002). However, rescue helicopters are not suitable means of transport during current thunderstorm situations, as they can be struck by lightning and crash (Cherington 1995; Zafren et al. 2005). As a means of communication, first responders can safely use mobile phones and other cordless phones. On the other hand, corded phones should be avoided as there have been severe injuries while making phone calls in the past (Andrews 1992; Dinakaram et al. 1998).

As a lightning strike accident that occurred in 2016 in Kentucky (USA), injuring two paramedics during their response to a traffic accident, demonstrates, the need for self-protection for first responders in thunderstorm situations is not only necessary for the emergency medical care of lightning victims, but for all potential operations (Leitchfield 2016).

▶ **Note** In the rescue of victims struck by lightning, self-protection has priority.

5.2 Triage

In about 30% of all fatal lightning accidents, there are other injured persons, with the clinical symptoms and injury patterns varying greatly (Whitcomb et al. 2002). The peculiarity in lightning accidents, however, is that the recognized triage rules for different types of trauma patients do not apply to victims of a lightning strike with subsequent cardiac and respiratory arrest. In a lightning accident, the resuscitation measures of injured persons without vital functions have absolute priority. The medical care of lightning victims with preserved vital functions is provided in every lightning accident only after the initial care of the apparently lifeless (Cooper 1992; Hinkelbein et al. 2013; Lederer et al. 2002; Association of Electrical Engineering Electronics Information Technology 2012; Zafren et al. 2005). This deviation from the recognized triage rules for trauma patients arises, among other things, from the numerous case reports of long-term successful resuscitations after lightning strikes and the knowledge that injured persons without primary respiratory or cardiac arrest usually do not develop life-threatening conditions in the next minutes to hours (Cooper 1980; Diepenseifen et al. 2009; Duppel et al. 2009; Hey and Rieder 1983; Holle et al. 2021; Lederer et al. 2002; Roesener 1962; Thompson et al. 2017; Zack et al. 1997).

> **Note** While in a different type of accident with a mass casualty incident, the victims with recognizable signs of life are given the first attention, the first treatment measures in a group of lightning strike victims are always to be carried out on the apparently lifeless victims with respiratory and/or circulatory arrest.

5.3 Lay Aid and Preclinical Emergency Medicine

5.3.1 Severity of Injuries

The consequences of a lightning strike can be very diverse for victims. After a lightning accident, people can either die immediately or after a latency period of hours, days or weeks, or they can survive the lightning strike. Among the survivors, there can either be a complete recovery, transient or persistent health damage (Backhaus et al. 2016; Cooper 1992; Ebertz 1891; Lichtenberg et al. 1993; Muehlberger et al. 2001; Umminger 2018; Zack et al. 2007, 2009, 2013). The American emergency physician Cooper (1992) divided the injured victims into three severity levels and defined these still unchallenged levels as follows:

1. *Mildly injured*
   The mildly injured patient is awake immediately after the lightning strike, slightly confused and can answer questions. He may have amnesia for the accident and difficulties with short-term memory for a few hours or days after the incident. Mildly injured patients sometimes complain of temporary hearing loss or visual disturbances, but rarely show skin burns. They may experience a usually unilateral tympanic membrane rupture due to the explosive bang.
   Vital functions are usually stable. A victim may occasionally exhibit temporary mild hypertension, which in most cases does not require treatment. Recovery usually occurs gradually.
   Injured individuals sometimes complain of paresthesias and/or muscle pain, which can persist for several weeks or months.
2. *Moderately injured*
   The moderately injured patient may be disoriented or comatose. Victims often have paralysis of the lower and/or upper extremities, which lasts several hours. The affected limbs appear cyanotic, speckled, pale, and pulseless. Differential diagnosis to hypovolemic shock is sometimes not easy. If hypotension is present, the patient should be examined for spinal injuries and other shock causes such as blunt abdominal injuries or fractures. First and second degree burns may be present. Tympanic membrane injuries are common. Moderately injured individuals may have suffered a temporary cardiopulmonary arrest due to the lightning strike and recover spontaneously. They should receive ECG examinations. In rare cases, these victims may experience seizures. Moderately injured individuals have a high probability of survival.

However, they may also develop permanent sequelae such as sleep disorders, paresthesias, general weakness, motor disorders, personality changes and/or cognitive disorders.

3. *Severely injured*
   Severely injured victims usually suffer a cardiac arrest with asystole or ventricular fibrillation, so resuscitation measures are required. While there are case reports in the literature about survival after prolonged resuscitation, there is no reason to assume that a positive outcome is the norm. Victims in this group may have direct brain damage caused by the lightning strike, hypoxic brain damage as a result of asystole, ventricular fibrillation or respiratory arrest, but also blunt traumas with intracranial injuries. The prognosis for recovery of victims in this group is rather unfavorable, except for the severely injured who respond quickly to resuscitation measures.

5.3.2 Causes of Respiratory and/or Cardiac Arrest

The causes of a respiratory and/or cardiac arrest following a lightning strike accident can be damage to the medullary respiratory center or the heart. The immediate effect on the heart can manifest as asystole or ventricular fibrillation. It is possible that after the accident, the heart action may spontaneously resume or only start after resuscitation measures. In contrast to the sometimes only briefly occurring asystole, a respiratory arrest caused by a lightning strike can last longer and thus also lead to a secondary hypoxic cardiac arrest (Fontanorosa 1993). The phenomenon described in the literature that victims of lightning strikes with respiratory and/or cardiac arrest have survived without subsequent damage even after delayed resuscitation measures (many minutes) is not yet clarified. However, this phenomenon leads to the recommendation to always start cardiopulmonary resuscitation treatment even after an unknown period of respiratory and/or cardiac arrest and in the absence of certain signs of death (livor mortis, rigor mortis) (Cooper et al. 2001; Cooper and Holle 2019; Hey and Rieder 1983; Holle et al. 2021; Lederer et al. 2002).

5.3.3 Basic Measures by Lay Helpers

Since there have been repeated severe accidents in the past when making a phone call with a corded telephone during thunderstorm conditions, accident witnesses or finders should always use a mobile phone or a cordless phone when making an emergency call, as these are considered safe (Andrews 1992; Lederer et al. 2002; Mahajan et al. 2008).

A large proportion of lightning accidents occur outdoors outside large cities, so many minutes, or under unfavorable circumstances even more than an hour, can pass until the arrival of the emergency doctor and other rescue services. Therefore, the chance of a successful resuscitation is usually only possible through an early start of Basic Life

Support by witnesses of the accident or finders (Hey and Rieder 1983; Lederer et al. 2002; Spano et al. 2015).

A victim of a lightning strike can suffer a range of injuries, from mild dizziness to immediate respiratory and/or cardiac arrest. Therefore, lay help on site must take into account the severity of the injuries (Cooper 1980). In accidents with several injured people, it also applies to first responders that help for the apparently lifeless victims has absolute priority, while extinguishing a strongly burning clothing of a living victim is by no means secondary (McCrady-Kahn and Kahn 1981).

According to the guidelines of the European Resuscitation Council for cardiopulmonary resuscitation, basic measures begin with checking for response and breathing (a missing pulse is obsolete as a criterion), followed by alerting the rescue service and starting chest compressions and ventilations in a 30:2 ratio ("Check—Call—Compress"). If a mobile phone is available, the speaker and hands-free function of the phone should be activated and cardiopulmonary resuscitation should be carried out with the support of the emergency call center. If possible, another helper should bring an automated external defibrillator and apply it. Uninterrupted chest compression has the highest priority, as any even brief interruption of chest compression is associated with a temporary cessation of organ perfusion and thus an intensification of ischemia, which in this situation is particularly threatening for the brain (risk of hypoxic brain damage) (Cherington 1995; Michels et al. 2022; Zack et al. 1997).

The location of the start of cardiopulmonary resuscitation measures for a victim of a lightning strike should ideally be relatively safe, e.g., a closed house or a vehicle with a metal body. Since a large proportion of lightning accidents occur outdoors in rural areas or in the mountains, this will often not be possible in practice (Elsom and Webb 2014; Harms 1956; Walsh et al. 2013).

Case Study

In July 1982, a 36-year-old woman in Baden-Württemberg (Germany) was struck by lightning at a barbecue area under a tree. The husband, who according to witnesses was only briefly unconscious after this lightning strike, began, assisted by the witnesses, to perform mouth-to-mouth resuscitation and chest compressions on the lifeless woman. Upon the arrival of the paramedics about 15 minutes after the lightning strike, the woman was in asystole and had wide, unresponsive pupils. After intubation, continuation of chest compressions, infusion therapy (sodium bicarbonate and dexamethasone), sinus tachycardia with a systolic blood pressure of 80 mmHg was detected after 10 minutes. After the arrival of the emergency doctor, administration of dopamine and transport to a city hospital.

Admission findings: Second-degree burns on the right temple, neck, and chest, coma, no spontaneous breathing, miosis, no corneal reflexes, blood pressure: 140/70 mmHg, heart rate: 120/min, ECG: flattened T-wave in V5 and V6, leukocytosis, hypokalemia, and increases in the serum concentrations of CK and glutamate-oxaloacetate transaminase (GOT).

Clinical course: Onset of spontaneous breathing after one day and extubation after 2 days, highly fluctuating level of consciousness until the 5th day, then clear consciousness, locally oriented, temporally disoriented, retrograde amnesia, signs of a cerebellar lesion (ataxia, dysmetria, dysdiadochokinesis), hypotonia of the skeletal muscles, pneumonia, successful mobilization, cooperation with neurologists, improvement of most pathological findings.

Discharge findings about 4 weeks after the accident: Short-term memory disorders, able to walk on her own despite still existing ataxia, ECG: T-wave inversion.

Conclusion of the authors: It can be assumed that without immediate lay help, this relatively good course would not have been possible (Hey and Rieder 1983). ◀

▶ **Note** In comparison to other types of accidents, there are some special particularities for rescue measures at the scene of a lightning strike with personal injury (see following overview).

5.3.4 Advanced Measures by Qualified Personnel

Upon the arrival of qualified rescue personnel, considering self-protection in the case of multiple injuries and a limitation of personnel and equipment, the monitoring of vital functions must be limited to unconscious individuals and advanced life-saving measures must be initiated immediately. It can be assumed that a life-threatening situation is not to be expected in all non-unconscious victims of a lightning strike (Cooper 1980; Lederer et al. 2002). A victim of a lightning strike who is breathing and speaking has a very good prognosis for survival of the accident and should be examined and treated in a clinic depending on symptoms, if cardiac, neurological, otological, ophthalmological damage or burns are apparent or considered (Hinkelbein et al. 2013; Lederer et al. 2002; Zafren et al. 2005). For the victims who are immediately taken over by lay helpers during ongoing basic measures, pulse oximetry, ECG recordings and defibrillation should be performed if indicated. After successful intubation to secure the airways, ventilation should be performed. In this context, it must be mentioned that several case reports have described aspiration of vomit shortly after the accident with subsequent aspiration pneumonia as the cause of death in victims of lightning strikes (Hanson and McIllwraith 1973; McCrady-Kahn and Kahn 1981; Möhle et al. 2015). In the case of ongoing lightning danger, manual ventilation is preferable to machine ventilation (Lederer et al. 2002).

After establishing an intravenous access, case-related drug therapy (vasopressors, antiarrhythmics, analgesics, sedatives, fluid replacement etc.) should be initiated. If there is no accident-related hypovolemia, volume substitution should be carried out with restraint (Lederer et al. 2002). If indicated, an external pacemaker should be used. It is known that implanted pacemakers can malfunction after a lightning strike (Obszanski 2019). Furthermore, case-related treatment such as the application of bandages for burns and bleeding, immobilization of fractures, and thermal protection should be carried out.

Due to the special situation of lightning strike accidents involving people, a termination of resuscitation measures should only be considered if no spontaneous circulation has occurred even after one hour of resuscitation treatment (Lederer et al. 2002).

Special Features in First Aid and Advanced Assistance after a Lightning Accident with Personal Injury

- First think of self-protection
- In case of multiple injuries, first help victims without signs of life
- Make emergency calls with cordless phones
- Prefer manual ventilation in case of ongoing lightning strike danger
- Consider terminating unsuccessful resuscitation treatment only after one hour

5.4 Transport

The subsequent care of lightning strike victims is carried out in consultation with the control center or other coordination points (Liebold et al. 2022). The destination of the transport of the victims depends on the type and severity of the injuries. Outpatient treatment is sufficient for minor injuries (Diepenseifen et al. 2009; Cooper 1980). For moderately and severely injured patients, inpatient monitoring and therapy are indicated. The targeted transport is based on the care options of the individual clinics. Severely injured patients should generally be taken to a maximum care hospital, e.g., university hospitals, to be treated in an intensive care unit. As soon as burns are the main concern, a center for severe burn injuries is preferred (Hinkelbein et al. 2013).

Case Study

On August 12, 2015, at around 4:45 pm, a lightning strike into a tree injured 44 military personnel who were in the immediate vicinity for their training in Florida (USA). The victims were triaged on site by the medical service, which had arrived by rescue helicopter immediately after the alarm was raised. It was estimated that 20 of the affected 44 recruits should receive inpatient monitoring or treatment. One man, who had suffered a cardiac arrest and had a Glasgow Coma Score of 6 at the time of triage, was transported to the emergency department of the responsible Air Base with two other injured recruits by rescue helicopter, where they arrived at 5:14 pm. All other injured persons were brought to the same emergency department by ambulance, private cars, and the returned rescue helicopter. The man who survived the cardiac arrest and 2 other victims were admitted to an intensive care unit. The other 17 injured were admitted to a regular ward for observation, e.g., due to cardiac arrhythmias. All 44 military personnel, including the patients from the intensive care unit, were discharged without restrictions one day after the lightning strike and were allowed to resume service under increased medical supervision (Thompson et al. 2017). ◀

References

Andrews CJ (1992) Telephon related lightning injury. Med J Australia 157:823–828

Backhaus R, Kirzinger L, Platen S, Kreuzer PM, Kleiter I, Lürding R, Zack F, Schulte-Mattler W, Schalke B (2016) Blitzschlagverletzungen. Klin Neurophysiol 47:78–84

Cherington M (1995) Lightning and transportation. Semin Neurol 15:233–240

Cooper MA (1980) Lightning injuries: prognostic signs of death. Ann Emerg Med 9:134–138

Cooper MA (1992) Treatment of lightning injury. Introduction and first aid. In: Andrews CJ, Cooper MA, Darveniza M, Mackerras D (eds) Lightning injuries: electrical, medical, and legal aspects. CRC Press, Boca Raton, pp 117–119

Cooper MA, Holle RL (2019) Reducing lightning injuries worldwide. Springer, Cham

Cooper MA, Andrews CJ, Holle RL, Lopez RE (2001) Lightning injuries. In: Auerbach PS (ed) Wilderness Medicine. 4th edn. Mosby, St. Louis, pp 73–110

Diepenseifen CJ, Schewe JC, Malotki F, Conrad H (2009) Blitzunfall bei Flugschau. Notfall Rettungsmed 12:523–530

Dinakaran S, Desai SP, Elsom DM (1998) Telephone-mediated lightning injury causing cataract. Injury 29:645–646

Duppel H, Löbermann M, Reisinger EC (2009) Aus heiterem Himmel vom Blitz getroffen. Dtsch Med Wochenschr 134:1214–1217

Ebertz M (1891) Ueber Blitzschlagverletzungen. Dtsch Med Wochenschr 36:1848–1852

Elsom DM, Webb JDC (2014) Deaths and injuries from lightning in the UK, 1988–2012. Weather 69:221–226

Fontanorosa PB (1993) Electric shock and lightning strike. Ann Emerg Med 22:378–387

Hanson GC, McIlwraith GR (1973) Lightning injury: two case histories and a review of management. Br Med J 4:271–274

Harms W (1956) Personenblitzschäden. Elektromedizin 1:153–158

Hey D, Rieder W (1983) Erfolgreiche Laien-Reanimation nach Blitzschlag. Dtsch Med Wochenschr 108:1217–1218

Hinkelbein J, Spelten O, Wetsch WA (2013) Blitzschlag und Blitzunfälle in der präklinischen Notfallmedizin. Unfallchirurg 116:74–79

Holle RL, Lopez RE, Howard KW, Vavrek J, Allsopp J (1995) Safety in the presence of lightning. Semin Neurol 15:375–380

Holle RL, Lopez RE, Zimmermann C (1999) Update recommendations for lightning safety. Bull Am Meteor Soc 80:2035–2041

Holle RL, Cooper MA, Navarrete-Aldana N (2021) Lightning injury: occurrence and medical treatment. In: Gomes C (ed) Lightning. Science, engineering, and economic implications for developing countries. Springer, Singapore, pp 263–273

Lederer W, Kroesen G (2005) Notfallmedizinische Versorgung von Blitz- und Stromschlagverletzungen. Anaesthesist 54:1120–1128

Lederer W, Wiedermann FJ, Baubin MA, Kroesen G (2002) Blitzschlagverletzung und kardiopulmonale Reanimation. Notfall & Rettungsmedizin 5:474–479

Leikin JB, Aks SE, Andrews S, Auerbach PS, Cooper MA, Jacobsen TD, Krenzelok EP, Shicker L, Weiner SL (1997) Environmental injuries. Dis Mon 43:809–816

Leitchfield K (2016) Lightning strike injures paramedic, EMT. https://www.ems1.com/trauma/articles/lightning-strike-injures-paramedic-emt-VBi3m2uNF5HhldJf/. Accessed: 13 Nov 2022.

Lichtenberg R, Dries D, Ward K, Marshall W, Scanlon P (1993) Cardiovascular effects of lightning strikes. J Am Coll Cardiol 21:531–536

Liebold F, Adams NB, Hinkelbein J (2022) Strom- und Blitzunfälle im Rettungsdienst. Notfallmedizin up2date. 17:423–440

Mackerras D (1992) Protection from lightning. In: Andrews CJ, Cooper MA, Darveniza M, Mackerras D (eds) Lightning injuries: electrical, medical, and legal aspects. CRC Press, Boca Raton, pp 145–156

Mahajan AL, Rajan R, Regan PJ (2008) Lichtenberg figures: cutaneous manifestation of phone electrocution from lightning. J Plast Reconstr Aesthet Surg 61:111–113

McCrady-Kahn VL, Kahn AM (1981) Lightning burns. West J Med 134:215–219

Michels G, Bauersachs J, Böttiger BW, Busch HJ, Dirks B, Frey N, Lott C, Rott N, Schöls W, Schulze PC, Thiele H (2022) Leitlinien des European Resuscitation Council (ERC) zur kardiopulmonalen Reanimation 2021: Update und Kommentar. Kardiologe 16:22–33

Möhle F, Preuss J, Madea B, Doberentz E (2015) Vier Tage überlebter Blitzschlag nach zunächst erfolgreicher Reanimation. Rechtsmedizin 25:561–565

Muehlberger T, Vogt PM, Munster AM (2001) The long-term consequences of lightning injuries. Burns 27:829–833

Obszanski B, Tulecki L, Kutarski A, Kleinrok A (2019) Lightning-induced pacing system malfunction: a case report. Eur Heart J Cas Rep 3:1–5

Rakov VA, Uman MA (2006) Lightning physics and effects. Cambridge University Press, Cambridge New York Melbourne Madrid Cape Town Singapore Sao Paulo

Roesener G (1962) Klinische und elektrokardiographische Beobachtungen an sechs durch Blitzschlag getroffenen Menschen. Elektromedizin 7:24–34

Spano SJ, Campagne D, Stroh G, Shalit M (2015) A lightning multiple casuality incident in Sequoia and Kings Canyon National Parks. Wilderness Environ Med 26:43–53

Stütz N, Weiss D, Reichert B (2006) Verletzungen durch Blitzschlag. Unfallchirurg 109:495–498

Thompson SN, Wilson ZW, Cole CB, Kennedy AR, Aycock RD (2017) Case report: mass casuality lightning strike at ranger training camp. Mil Med 182:e1803–e1806

Uman MA (1986) All about lightning. Dover Publications, New York

Umminger JM (2018) Neurologische Langzeitschäden bei Blitzopfern—vergleichende Literaturrecherche zu neurologischen, neuropsychologischen und psychiatrischen Langzeitschäden nach Blitzschlag, deren Behandlung und Prognose. Med Diss. Universität Regensburg, Regensburg

Verband der Elektrotechnik Elektronik Informationstechnik e. V. (2012) Unfälle durch Blitzeinwirkung. https://www.vde.com/resource/blob/936982/0f4076543f8f7ec91e3774536ca17ee0/merkblatt-blitzunfaelle-download-data.pdf. Accessed: 27 Jan 2020.

Walsh KM, Cooper MA, Holle R, Rakov VA, Roeder WP, Ryan M (2013) National Athletic Trainers' Association position statement: lightning safety for athletics and recreation. J Athl Train 48:258–270

Whitcomb D, Martinez JA, Daberkow D (2002) Lightning injuries. South Med J 95:1331–1334

Zack F, Hammer U, Klett I, Wegener R (1997) Myocardial injury due to lightning. Int J Legal Med 110:326–328

Zack F, Rothschild MA, Wegener R (2007) Blitzunfall—Energieübertragungsmechanismen und medizinische Folgen. Dtsch Ärztebl 104:A3545–A3549

Zack F, Rummel J, Püschel K (2009) Blitzschläge auf Fußballplätzen. Eine unterschätzte Gefahr. Rechtsmedizin 19:77–82

Zack F, Raphael T, Kupfer J, Jokuszies A, Vogt PM, Büttner A, Püschel K, Schalke B, Todt M, Dettmeyer R (2013) Vier Todesopfer nach einem Blitzunfall auf einem Golfplatz. Rechtsmedizin 23:114–118

Zafren K, Durrer B, Herry JP, Brugger H, ICAR MEDCOM, UIAA MEDCOM (2005) Lightning injuries: prevention and on-site treatment in mountains and remote areas. Official guidelines of the International Commission for Mountain Emergency Medicine and the Medical Commission of the International Mountaineering and Climbing Federation. Resuscitation 65:369–372

Zimmermann C, Cooper MA, Holle RL (2002) Lightning safety guidelines. Ann Emerg Med 39:660–664

Clinical Medicine

6

6.1 Diagnosis

6.1.1 Diagnosis of Lightning Strike Accidents

The establishment of the diagnosis *Injuries due to lightning strike* is in the majority of cases not a difficult task, as the accident has either been witnessed or multiple injured persons have occurred at an event. On the other hand, unwitnessed accidents of individual persons can indeed pose problems in terms of diagnosis (Cherington et al. 2001; Schaidt 1977; Sellier 1975). In contrast to the lethal accident, where the coroner can consider the simultaneously deceased animals, the crater in the ground, or damaged objects in the immediate vicinity of the accident site for his overall assessment, treating physicians in the clinic often receive sparse or no information about the location where the patient was found (see Chap. 7). Initial treating physicians, who get to see the clothing worn by the victim at the time of the accident, can gain valuable clues for the correct diagnosis from tears, caused by the explosive pressure wave at the accident site. However, the findings that have the highest relevance for the diagnosis *Injuries due to lightning strike* are located on the body surface and can be determined by a simple inspection under good lighting conditions. Singeing of body hair is considered pathognomonic for exposure to lightning strike (Blumenthal 2005; Jellinek 1903). These curled, mostly blackish hair changes occur especially on the head, chest, abdominal, pubic hair and legs (Fig. 6.1) and are found much more frequently than Lichtenberg figures (Blumenthal 2005; Bremer 2024). The Lichtenberg figures, which are also considered pathognomonic for the diagnosis of lightning strike injury, have two disadvantages compared to the singed hair. On the one hand, they do not persist after the accident, but fade and disappear within hours to days (Table 7.1) (Zack and Büttner 2016). On the other hand, they are extremely rarely detectable in dark-skinned victims (Blumenthal 2005; Dutta

F. Zack, *Accidents Caused by Lightning Strikes*,
https://doi.org/10.1007/978-3-662-71066-1_6

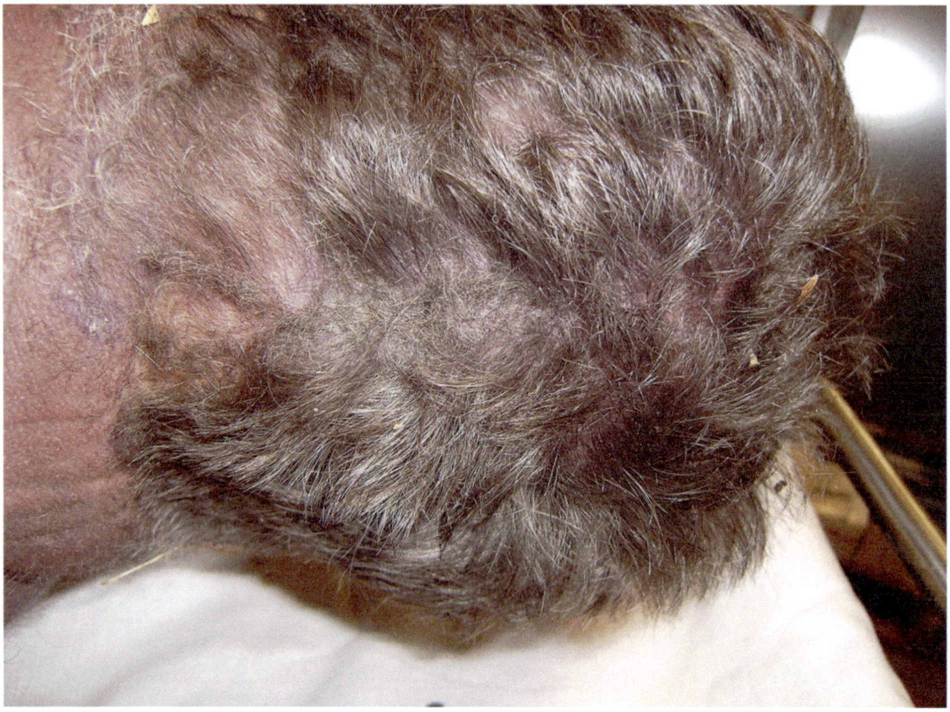

Fig. 6.1 Singed hair, here on the back of a man's head, is considered pathognomonic for an accident due to lightning strike. (Own illustration)

2016). But also other lightning strike-related changes on the patient's body surface, such as burns of various types or metallization effects (see Chap. 7) can lead the doctors to the correct diagnosis. In rare cases, however, there were also lightning strike accidents that caused no characteristic external findings. For these cases, the magnetic field existing around a lightning bolt is preferably held responsible (Cherington et al. 1998; Zack et al. 1997). In clarifying such accidents, the responsible regional lightning detection systems of the countries can help (see Chap. 3 and Table 7.3). With the support of these modern systems, any interested person can inquire whether one or more lightning strikes have been registered for the period shortly before the discovery of a victim of an unwitnessed accident and the event location (Cherington et al. 1997, 2001; Kleiter et al. 2007; Püschel et al. 2009; Zack et al. 2013).

In making the correct diagnosis, a severely injured victim (see chap. 5) can almost never actively assist, as it usually has a retrograde amnesia that includes the time of the accident.

Once the diagnosis of *injuries caused by lightning strike* is confirmed, the first part of the diagnosis has been completed.

6.1.2 Principles of Diagnosing Individual Health Damages

The second part of the diagnosis involves determining the individual injuries of the patients and the subsequent damages. This task can be just as problematic for the treating physicians, as there is no uniform injury pattern in humans after a lightning accident, but on the contrary, the health damages show a great variety.

From this expertise, two principles for the diagnosis and therapy of severely injured lightning strike victims emerge:

- Since lightning strikes can cause numerous different injuries to organs or organ systems, intensivists should involve colleagues from other disciplines (e.g., cardiologists, neurologists, ophthalmologists, ENT doctors, surgeons, psychologists) in the diagnosis and therapy of severely injured patients at an early stage.
- As part of the diagnosis, an attempt should always be made to reconstruct the mechanism of energy transfer to the victim, as this path has an influence on the expected injuries. For example, lightning-traumatic myocardial necroses often occurred after direct hits (see chap. 4) that were survived (Hanson and McIlwraith 1973; van Ruler et al. 2022; Zack et al. 1997). After damage caused by a barotrauma, injuries to the hearing organ and the cranial-brain region were repeatedly detected (Angerer et al. 2009; Blumenthal 2021; Just et al. 2002; Murty 2009).

The diagnosis and therapy as well as the outcome of the individual injuries are dealt with in the following sections, sorted by organs and organ systems.

Specifics of Making The Diagnosis *Injuries Caused by Lightning Strike*

- Clarifying the diagnosis is straightforward in observed cases and events with multiple victims.
- Difficulties may arise in recognizing the correct cause of injuries when the accident has not been observed.
- Inspection of the body surface and the clothing worn leads to the correct diagnosis in the majority of cases.
- In unclear cases, it is recommended to consult the records of the responsible regional lightning detection system.
- After a lightning strike accident, there is no uniform injury pattern for a human victim.
- Knowledge of the energy transfer mechanism at the accident site can provide clues to the expected injury pattern for a specific case.
- The diagnosis of severely injured patients should always be interdisciplinary.

6.2 Diagnosis of Early and Late Effects, Therapy, Outcome

The following sections focus on the diagnosis and therapy of particularly moderately and severely injured lightning victims, because apparently lightly injured patients either do not need to be hospitalized or can be discharged after a few hours of monitoring.

Especially in the case of severely injured patients, diagnosis, therapy, and prognostic predictions immediately after the patient is taken over by the rescue service are extremely problematic. This is due to the fact that only extremely few doctors have experience in treating lightning strike victims, and also because almost no lightning accident is like any other.

The health damage caused by a lightning strike in an accident is not evenly distributed among the individual organs and organ systems. For example, while the pancreas, spleen, and sexual organs are very rarely affected, lightning strikes relatively frequently injure the skin, heart, central and peripheral nervous system, and the auditory and visual organs. The consequences of a lightning strike can be divided into four categories in terms of their temporal occurrence (Cherington 2003):

- immediate and temporary,
- immediate or prolonged occurrence or persistence,
- delayed occurrence with often progressive course,
- occurrence is possible at any time.

The following presents injuries and long-term effects frequently observed in individuals after a lightning accident.

6.2.1 Skin

Not every victim of a lightning strike shows signs of burns or Lichtenberg figures. While Cooper (1980) found burns in 36 of 54 (66%) injured people who had to be hospitalized, Holle et al. (2021) report that less than a third of all lightning strike victims show changes in the skin. In contrast to accidents caused by technical high voltage, where deep burns often occur, burns caused by lightning strikes are predominantly on the skin. If the high temperatures of the lightning's plasma channel do not lead to an open fire at the accident site, the extent of the injured body surface is no more than 20% (Table 6.1). However, if clothing or objects in the vicinity catch fire, burns covering 70% of the body surface have been described (Ventura et al. 2017). Thus, some victims of lightning strikes are eligible for immediate transport from the accident site or emergency room to a burn center. In the current guideline of the German Society for Burn Medicine (2021, AWMF register no.: 044-001) on the *treatment of thermal injuries in adults*, lightning accidents are not listed under electrical accidents or under a separate point. However, the considerable differences

Table 6.1 Extent of burns to the body surface after a lightning strike. (Own representation)

Burn injuries to the body surface in %	Authors	Age (years)	Gender	Special features	Degree of burn	Outcome
3.5	Sleihwah et al. 2018	5	m	n. s.	n. s.	Survived
4,5	Lakshminarayanan et al. 2009	39	m	n. s.	n. s.	Survived
6	Tadler et al. 2017	75	f	Shoe smoked	1 to 2	Survived
10	Ozgun and Castillo 1995	32	m	n. s.	n. s.	Survived
10	Koeppen 1965	44	m	n. s.	n. s.	Deceased
10	Spaar 1955	44	m	Clothing burned	3	Deceased
11	Stütz et al. 2006	17	m	n. s.	2	Survived
20	Hawkes and Thorpe 1992	19	m	n. s.	n. s.	Survived
20	Kilbas et al. 2008	22	m	n. s.	n. s.	Deceased
23	Amy et al. 1985	16	m	Clothing caught fire	3	Survived
31	McCrady-Kahn and Kahn 1981	10	m	Clothing caught fire	n. s.	Survived
70	Ventura et al. 2017	53	m	Clothing caught fire	1 to 3	Deceased

m male, f female, n. s. not specified

between an accident caused by technical electricity and a lightning strike are shown by the difficult-to-compare accident situations and the sometimes different consequences. For example, acute renal failure due to an acute tubulopathy after a lightning accident, unlike an accident caused by technical high voltage, is extremely rare (Cooper et al. 2017).

For the diagnosis of burns after a lightning strike, a careful inspection of the entire unclothed body surface is usually sufficient. Of the variety of possible skin injuries, large-area burns from igniting clothing, apart from damage to other organs, are most likely life-threatening (Ventura et al. 2017).

Even if the accident caused by lightning strike has not yet been explicitly included in the specified AWMF guideline, the treatment of burns requiring treatment should also be carried out according to this guideline after a lightning accident. This includes recommendations for preclinical measures, transfer and admission to a clinic for burn-injured adults, trauma room management, analgosedation, intensive medical therapy of the shock phase, ventilation, nutrition, anti-infective therapy, pain treatment, care of the burn wound, psychological therapy, rehabilitation and treatment of the consequences of burns (German Society for Burn Medicine 2021, AWMF register no.: 044-001).

In contrast to severely injured patients due to a technical high-voltage accident, the prognosis for patients with isolated skin damage after a lightning strike is predominantly good. In these patients, scars or tattoo-like metallization effects can remain due to evaporated necklaces (Jonas et al. 2002; Stütz et al. 2006). However, injuries to other organs or organ systems often occur after a lightning strike accident, which can then determine the prognosis (Cooper et al. 2017; Schniers 2005).

Case Study

During a football match in Bavaria (Germany), a summer storm arose, and lightning struck the field. Of the numerous players, only one person was injured. The teammates buried the injured 17-year-old man, except for his head, in wet sand and alerted the emergency services. The emergency doctor intubated the man at the scene of the accident. Upon arrival at a center for severe burn injuries, the football player had a 6 cm long, open skin injury on the right side of his neck and second-degree burns covering 11% of his body surface on his chest, abdomen, and both lower legs. The subsequent clinical examinations including ECG, echocardiography, and sonography of the abdomen showed no pathological findings. X-ray diagnostics of the thorax, axial skeleton, and pelvis revealed no signs of fractures. The man complained of visual disturbances, which had been caused by conjunctival irritation. After local administration of an antibiotic for 4 days, the symptoms subsided. After the insertion of a central venous catheter, fluid replacement was carried out. At the time of admission, the laboratory parameters creatine kinase (CK), myoglobin and C-reactive proteinin the serum were elevated (Table 6.2).

On the day of the accident, the wounds were cleaned under anesthesia and the burn wounds were treated with sterile dressings. Extubation was performed one day after the accident. On the 3rd day of inpatient treatment, a necrosectomy was performed on the right lower leg and the area was covered with split skin. In the same session, the open neck wound was closed using a Z-plasty. The postoperative wound healing process was uncomplicated. All laboratory parameters were within the normal range on

Table 6.2 Laboratory parameters on the day of the 17-year-old accident victim's hospital admission. (Own representation)

Laboratory parameter	Serum concentration	Reference range
CK	720 U/l	<170 U/l
CK-MB	18.1 U/l	<25 U/l
Myoglobin	749.1 µg/l	23–72 µg/l
C-reactive protein	8.9 mg/dl	0.5 mg/dl
Troponin	0.06 µg/l	<0.4 µg/l

the 4th day after the accident. The onset of a post-traumatic stress reaction, which the patient developed, was not dated. This consequence of the accident could be reduced by psychological support during the inpatient stay, which lasted 14 days. The further course of the post-traumatic stress reaction is not reported in the case study (Stütz et al. 2006).

This case is also noteworthy in that the historical recommendation from *The New Healing Method,* to bury an injured person after a lightning strike accident, except for the head, was still being applied almost 100 years later (Platen 1913). Whether the additional sandy contamination of the skin injuries prolonged wound healing is not mentioned in the case study.

In addition to burns, a lightning strike can cause other effects on a person's skin. Netchiporouk et al. (2015) report on a 17-year-old man who initially had 2nd-3rd degree burns on his skin and developed eruptive disseminated pyogenic granulomas in and outside the thermally damaged skin about 2 weeks after the accident. ◀

Characteristics of Skin Injuries from Lightning Strikes

- Victims of lightning strikes usually exhibit superficial burns of varying shape and location, which generally do not exceed 20% of the body surface area.
- Lightning strikes can set a victim's clothing on fire, which can, albeit rarely, lead to life-threatening burns to the body surface.
- Some victims of lightning strikes may be considered for immediate transport from the accident site or emergency room to a burn center.
- Superficial skin injuries usually heal without complications.
- In the case of deeper injuries, plastic surgical treatment will usually be required.

6.2.2 Cardiovascular System

The effects of a lightning strike on the cardiovascular system are diverse, depending on the energy transfer mechanisms, and range from minor ECG changes to sudden death.

The human cardiovascular system is often affected in accidents caused by lightning strikes. After a direct hit or a side flash, asystole or ventricular fibrillation often occur, and after successful resuscitation measures, tachycardia, hypertension, anginal complaints, and/or lightning-induced myocardial necrosis may occur (Apfelberg et al. 1974; Cooper and Holle 2019; Davis et al. 2014; Hanson and McIlwraith 1973; Lichtenberg et al.1993; Zack et al. 1997, 2007). The following presents both common and only occasionally observed effects of a lightning strike accident on the human cardiovascular system.

6.2.2.1 Cardiac Arrhythmias

Numerous case reports describe different cardiac arrhythmias after a lightning strike accident. The question of which arrhythmias of the heartbeat occur immediately after the event is difficult to answer, as victims usually do not have a long-term electrocardiogram (ECG) at the time of the accident and the arrival of emergency medical rescue always occurs after a certain period of time. Thus, asystole or ventricular fibrillation are often detected when the first ECG is written at the accident site (Karobath et al. 1971; Koeppen 1965; Levy and Akiyama 2007; Lichtenberg et al. 1993; Wetli 1996). However, there are also reports that electromechanical dissociation or atrial fibrillation were documented after a lightning strike (Dronacahrya and Poudel 2008; Koeppen 1965; Leira et al. 2013; Levy and Akiyama 2007; Wetli 1996).

The exact pathophysiological backgrounds for the immediate asystole or ventricular fibrillation after a lightning strike are still not clarified today.

The causes for the acute cardiac arrest are seen on the one hand in the direct damage to the heart and on the other hand in a secondary consequence of a central respiratory arrest (Browne and Gaasch 1992; Cooper et al. 2001; Cooper and Holle 2019).

After successful resuscitation measures or survival without the need for resuscitation, victims of a lightning strike often exhibit sinus tachycardia (Lichtenberg et al. 1993).

6.2.2.2 Anginal Complaints and Lightning-Induced Myocardial Necrosis

After a lightning strike accident, a victim may develop pectoranginous complaints or a clinically diagnosed acute myocardial infarction in the following minutes to hours (Alyan et al. 2006; Dundon et al. 2008; Igbal et al. 2023; Kleinot et al. 1966; Sinha 1985; Zack et al. 1997; Zeana 1984). The underlying pathophysiological mechanisms for this are still unclear (see Chap. 7). Causes discussed include direct electrical damage, insufficient oxygen supply to the myocardium due to lack of filling of the coronary arteries, e.g., during persistent ventricular fibrillation until defibrillation, coronary spasms, lightning-induced stress, or disseminated intravascular coagulation (Ekoe et al. 1985; Geary et al. 2015; Schniers 2005; van Ruler et al. 2022). Coronary angiographies performed in connection with lightning-traumatic myocardial necroses, the results of which have been published in specialist articles, consistently showed unremarkable findings (Geary et al. 2015; Hayashi et al. 2005; Karadas et al. 2013). Therefore, the indication for a coronary angiography should generally be narrowly defined, especially in younger victims of a lightning strike. Infarction-typical pains, which are preferably located retrosternally but can also radiate, do not occur in every case (Sinha 1985). The patients show infarction-typical ECG changes, as are also observed in myocardial necroses due to severe coronary sclerosis. An increased troponin in the serum is not obligatory. Patients with lightning-induced myocardial infarctions usually survive the accident if they do not have any other life-threatening consequences (Table 6.3). The symptoms of myocardial infarction regress within days to weeks and at the time of hospital discharge, most victims are symptom-free. In patients who show other life-threatening accident conse-

Table 6.3 Published cases with myocardial infarction-like findings after surviving a lightning strike. (Own representation)

Age (years)	Gender	Time until the last check-up	Heart function limitations at hospital discharge	Authors
14	f	12 months	None	Burda 1966
20	f	n. s.	None	Kleinot et al. 1966
20	m	2 months	None	Sinha 1985
27	f	2 months	None	Eber et al. 1989
30	m	1 week	None	Kleinot et al. 1966
37	f	6 weeks	None	Dundon et al. 2008
38	m	1 month	None	Alyan et al. 2006
63	m	Self-discharge with persistent ECG changes after 3 weeks	None	Zeana 1984

m male, f female, n. s. not specified

quences in addition to lightning-traumatic myocardial necroses, the heart damage can contribute to a lethal course. However, in these tragic cases, hypoxic brain damage is in the foreground in terms of the cause of death (Table 6.4). With the exception of a rare indication for coronary angiography, diagnostics and monitoring should be carried out in accordance with guidelines (Werdan et al. 2021). In the treatment of a lightning-induced myocardial infarction, platelet aggregation inhibitors can be omitted (Aydin et al. 2018).

Case Study

A 20-year-old man in India was struck by lightning and presented with retrosternal pain in a clinic about 30 h later. Upon admission, an agitated, slightly dehydrated patient with a sinus tachycardia of 120 beats/min and a blood pressure of 86/60 mmHg was noticed. The victim had superficial skin burns on the face, chest, abdomen, and both anterior thighs, predominantly of the 2nd degree. The ECG taken on admission showed a negative T-wave in leads II, III, aVF, V3, and V4, as well as ST-segment elevation in V3 and V4. Immediate therapy was initiated with intravenous fluid replacement, administration of an analgesic, antibiotic, long-acting glucocorticoid, and treatment of the burns.

On the 2nd day after hospital admission, the clinical condition stabilized and the blood pressure was 110/72 mmHg. However, the patient continued to complain of retrosternal pain. The ECG taken on this day showed deep negative T-waves in leads II, III, aVF, and V2-V5, and continued ST-segment elevations in V2 and V3. The diagnosis of an acute myocardial infarction induced by lightning strike, particularly of the

Table 6.4 Published cases of lightning-induced myocardial necrosis/acute myocardial infarction following a briefly survived lightning strike accident. (Own representation)

Age (Years)	Gender	Survival Time	Main Cause of Death	Authors
8	m	3 Days	Hypoxic Brain Damage	Harwood et al. 1978
9	m	12 h	Aspiration Pneumonia	Hanson and McIlwraith 1973
9	m	7 Days	Hypoxic Brain Damage	Kotagel et al. 1982
15	m	3 Days	Hypoxic Brain Damage	Wetli 1996
15	m	9 Days	Hypoxic Brain Damage	Hanson and McIlwraith 1973
15	m	10 Days	Multiorgan Failure	Kravitz et al. 1977
17	m	11 Days	Hypoxic Brain Damage	Schwab et al. 1989
21	m	20 h	Acute Myocardial Infarction	Aydin et al. 2018
24	f	24 h	Hypoxic brain damage	Ekoe et al. 1985
27	m	5 days	Hypoxic brain damage	Zack et al. 1997
44	m	24 h	Hypoxic brain damage	Karadas et al. 2013
55	m	4 days	Hypoxic brain damage	Whitcomb et al. 2002

m male, f female

anterior wall of the left ventricle, was made. The retrosternal pain was regressive due to the therapeutic measures.

The ECG taken on the 7th day of hospitalization showed a significant decrease in T-wave negativity and an inconspicuous ST-segment finding. The recovery was uncomplicated and the man was discharged from inpatient treatment in the 3rd week after the accident. A control ECG performed 2 months later showed only nonspecific T-wave changes (Sinha 1985). ◀

▶ **Note** In the case of myocardial necrosis due to lightning trauma, which clinically appears like an acute myocardial infarction, coronary angiography and therapy with platelet aggregation inhibitors can be omitted, especially in younger victims.

6.2.2.3 Ventricular Hypokinesia

A rare complication after a lightning strike accident is the development of Tako-Tsubo cardiomyopathy, also known as *stress cardiomyopathy* or *transient left ventricular apical ballooning,* which has been described in at least three female victims so far (Dundon et al. 2008; Hayashi et al. 2005; Tadler et al. 2017). Both ischemic and catecholamine-mediated cardiotoxic factors are discussed as causes. Hayashi et al. (2005) reported the first case in which a 62-year-old mountaineer was injured by a lightning strike in Japan, remained conscious, and due to the remote location of the accident, was not brought to a clinic by a rescue helicopter until 24 hours later. The echocardiography performed on the day of admission showed a tako-tsubo-like pattern of left ventricular hypokinesia. Furthermore, the ECG showed ST-segment elevation and T-wave inversion, the ejection fraction was 65% and the serum concentrations of the parameters CK, CK-MB and troponin were elevated. Based on these findings, the diagnosis of an acute myocardial infarction was made and the accident victim was treated with an analgesic and mononitrate. The coronary angiography showed no pathological findings. There was no heart failure and all pathological findings improved, so the woman could be discharged on the 11th day after hospital admission (Hayashi et al. 2005).

Significantly more severe disease courses were shown by two other female victims (37 and 75 years old) of a lightning strike with the development of the same complication. After treatment with an angiotensin-converting enzyme inhibitor and diuretic, the cardiac symptoms improved.

All women survived the accidents and showed no pathological findings of heart functions in follow-up examinations, which were carried out after 2, 4 and 6 weeks (Dundon et al. 2008; Tadler et al. 2017).

Lichtenberg et al. (1993) reported on a 36-year-old man who, after a direct hit in Illinois (USA), showed severe hypokinesia, particularly of the anterior wall of the heart, which was associated with ST-segment elevation in the ECG and an increase in the CK-MB concentration in the serum and completely regressed on the 4th day after the accident, so he could be discharged without complaints. Even though the diagnosis of Tako-Tsubo cardiomyopathy was not made in this case, it shows similarities to the accidents described above.

Kleiner and Wilkin (1978) reported on a lightning accident in the state of Georgia (USA), in which an 18-year-old man developed severe left ventricular dysfunction with the formation of pulmonary edema 3 hours after the event. After the start of diuretic therapy, there was an immediate improvement in symptoms. In control examinations, the heart still showed slight left ventricular hypokinesia with a reduction in the ejection fraction to 47% 6 weeks after the accident. A similar lightning strike accident, in which the symptoms in a 24-year-old woman were overcome after a week, was observed by Chia (1981) in Singapore. Nield and Kamat (2004) reported on a 10-year-old girl who showed global left ventricular dysfunction 2 days after a lightning strike accident in Michigan (USA), which quickly improved.

Case Study

A 37-year-old woman was struck by lightning in Australia as she ran from the beach to seek shelter from an approaching storm. She suffered an immediate cardiac arrest, which was resolved by quickly initiated resuscitation measures. Upon arrival at a clinic, she exhibited fluctuating levels of consciousness and complained of paresthesia of the extremities and face, as well as shoulder and back pain. She had contact burns on her neck from a worn chain and on her hip from rivets on her jeans. Her skin showed several Lichtenberg figures. The first clinical examination of the heart immediately after hospital admission was unremarkable. The admission ECG showed sinus tachycardia at 100 beats/min and slight ST-segment elevation in numerous leads. Shortly after admission, the patient developed pulmonary edema with dyspnea. Laboratory tests revealed elevated serum concentrations of the parameters CK, CK-MB, and Troponin T. The subsequent transthoracic echocardiography showed left ventricular apical akinesia and associated moderate to severe left ventricular systolic impairment despite preserved contractile function in the basal heart region. Based on these findings, the diagnosis of Tako-Tsubo cardiomyopathy was made. The subsequent ECG showed a striking anterolateral and inferior T-wave inversion, which was associated with ischemia of the myocardium. A coronary angiography performed 7 days later revealed no pathological findings. Therapy and monitoring focused on diuresis and heart monitoring. The patient was discharged after 6 weeks with fully recovered heart function (Dundon et al. 2008). ◀

6.2.2.4 Hypertension
Immediately after a lightning accident, hypertension often occurs, which regresses in the following hours and in the majority of cases does not need to be treated (Cooper 1995). The cause of this transient hypertension could be the keraunoparalysis often observed in accident victims, which is associated with vasoconstriction of the extremity vessels.

6.2.2.5 Hemorrhages
After a lightning strike, a victim's heart can develop extensive bleeding. These have been found intramyocardially, subendocardially and/or subepicardially and can have a diameter of several centimeters. The preferred location is the left ventricle. Depending on the size and location, such hemorrhages can cause different cardiac symptoms or remain symptomless. These bleedings are often only detected post-mortem during an autopsy (Blumenthal 2021; Möhle et al. 2015; Wetli 1996; Zack et al. 1997). While Wetli (1996) classified the described findings under Contusio cordis, the cause could be either a bruise or a rupture of intramyocardial vessels due to the barotrauma associated with the lightning strike (Blumenthal et al. 2012). According to the experience of forensic doctors, performed resuscitation measures are not suitable to explain such large bleedings in the mentioned locations (Buschmann and Tsokos 2008).

6.2.2.6 Pericarditis
Pericarditis following a lightning strike is a rare complication and has so far only occurred as a late consequence of an accident due to a combination of a direct hit, contact effect, and barotrauma.

Case Study

A 33-year-old woman in the state of Illinois (USA) was struck by lightning while carrying an open umbrella and was immediately admitted to a trauma center. The initial clinical examinations indicated thoracic and abdominal injuries. The patient had a sinus tachycardia with 124 beats/min and a systolic blood pressure of 80 mmHg. A performed peritoneal lavage revealed a significant amount of bloody-serous exudate. A subsequent laparotomy showed superficial injuries to the small and large intestines. After a windowing of the pericardium, about 200 ml of bloody-serous fluid was found in the pericardial sac. A drainage placed promoted another 800 ml of similar exudate over the next 24 hours. Within the first 8 hours after admission, the heart function deteriorated due to dilated and hypokinetic heart chambers on both sides. A radionuclide ventriculography showed a biventricular reduction in the ejection fraction. The administration of a synthetic sympathomimetic for inotropic support of the too low cardiac output led to an improvement in heart function. Three weeks after the accident, the patient was discharged from inpatient treatment and readmitted a week later with thoracic pain. Extensive cardiological diagnostics yielded no pathological findings. This was followed by cardiological rehabilitation treatment. After 3 and 5 months, the patient presented again with thoracic complaints, pericardial friction rub, and pericardial effusion. After therapy with oral steroids, the pericarditis regressed. At a follow-up visit after one year, the accident victim was symptom-free and showed no pathological findings in the echocardiography and magnetic resonance imaging (Lichtenberg et al. 1993). ◀

6.2.2.7 Pacemakers

A lightning accident can cause the subsequent malfunction of a patient's pacemaker due to electrical damage to the endocardial electrode interface. After a lightning strike, a transvenous electrode extraction may be required due to an acutely caused malfunction of the pacemaker (Obszanski et al. 2019).

▶ **Note** The function of a pacemaker should always be checked after an accident caused by a lightning strike.

6.2.2.8 ECG Changes

For all patients who have suffered a lightning strike, an early ECG is recommended (Kleiner and Wilkin 1978; Palmer 1987). The most common ECG changes observed in individuals after a lightning strike accident are elevation of the ST segment, T-wave inversion and a prolonged QTc interval (Burda 1966; Igbal et al. 2023; Lichtenberg et al. 1993; McIntyre et al. 2010; Palmer 1987; Tadler et al. 2017). In individual cases, other pathological findings such as an AV block 1. degree, right bundle branch block or widened QRS complex were also detected (Hawkes and Thorpe 1992; Mason and Crocett 2000; Tadler et al. 2017). After the occurrence of pathological ECG findings, the changes normalize in almost all cases in the first days and weeks after the accident (Palmer 1987; van Ruler et al. 2022).

6.2.2.9 Laboratory Parameters

The laboratory parameters that most frequently showed pathological findings in victims of a lightning accident with cardiac symptoms were the enzymes Creatine Kinase (CK) and CK-MB, as well as the muscle proteins Troponin I and T (Auer 2000; Harwood et al. 1978; Lichtenberg et al. 1993; Nield and Kamat 2004; Tadler et al. 2017). In contrast to the enzymes CK and CK-MB, which currently play no role in the diagnosis of an acute myocardial infarction, the cardiac muscle-specific biomarkers Troponin I and T are relevant for confirming the diagnosis (Herold and colleagues 2017).

6.2.2.10 Aorta

Three out of 45 deceased victims of a lightning accident showed injuries to the aorta, consisting of endothelial lesions, tears in the tunica media, and hemorrhages in the tunica adventitia. An aortic rupture as a result of a lightning strike has not been reported so far (Wetli 1996).

6.2.2.11 Therapy and Outcome

The therapy for cardiovascular complications of a lightning strike accident is carried out according to existing standards and guidelines, depending on the diagnosis. There is no guideline specifically related to a lightning strike accident.

Kleiner and Wilkin (1978) as well as Palmer (1987) generally recommend performing an ECG on every victim of a lightning strike. An indication for subsequent cardiac monitoring exists for patients who had to be resuscitated after the accident, show cardiac symptoms and/or have an abnormal ECG (Kirchmair and Dienstl 1982).

Approximately 8–27% of lightning strike victims die immediately or after a time interval due to the accident (see Chap. 7) (Puchstein 2016; Zack et al. 2016). It is currently assumed that in the majority of those who died at the accident site, the pathophysiological mechanisms asystole, ventricular fibrillation or central respiratory paralysis lead to death (Wetli 1996; Zack and Büttner 2020). In almost all accidents where the victims do not die at the scene, the not infrequently occurring cardiac complications are generally well survived. This also applies to lightning-induced myocardial necrosis/acute myocardial infarctions and transient cardiomyopathies. An exception are the intramyocardial hemorrhages, which have so far caused death after a time interval of 10 hours or 10 days in at least 2 cases (Blumenthal 2021; Wetli 1996). Except for one case where pericarditis was still detected 5 months after the lightning strike, the other cardiac complications have often been overcome without permanent damage after a few weeks (Lichtenberg et al. 1993).

Characteristic Cardiovascular Symptoms and Findings in Patients after Lightning Strike

- Immediate cardiac arrest, hypertension, tachycardia, and nonspecific ECG changes (ST-segment elevation, T-wave inversion, prolonged QTc interval) are common.
- Acute myocardial necrosis/myocardial infarctions, reduced left ventricular ejection fraction, and extensive myocardial bleeding are less common.
- The spontaneous return of circulation (Return Of Spontaneous Circulation—ROSC) is more the rule than the exception, but the respiratory arrest usually outlasts the cardiac arrest. Apnea is the critical factor for the outcome. Therefore, artificial ventilation must be continued after ROSC.
- ECG changes often occur with delays of hours and usually subside within a few days.
- Self-limiting vasospasms can mimic cardiac, gastrointestinal or neurological ischemia or even a compartment syndrome.
- Pacemakers can lose their functionality.

6.2.3 Central and Peripheral Nervous System

In survivors of lightning strike accidents, damage to the central and peripheral nervous systems are the most common long-term consequences. Once the lightning has overcome the human skin resistance, there is a very short current flow in the body. It particularly flows through tissues with a low electrical resistance, such as the nerves, and leaves, compared to technical high-voltage accidents, almost no severe internal burns. In principle, all parts of the central and peripheral nervous system can be affected (Cherington 2003). In addition to transient disturbances of consciousness and short-term limb paresis as well as sensory disturbances, structural lesions can also occur, particularly in the central nervous system (Cherington 2003; O'Keefe Gatewood and Zane 2004).

On the other hand, effects on the peripheral nervous system are less frequently documented. The occurrence of a variety of autonomic disorders and the particular sensitivity of non-myelinated nerve fibers strongly suggest that the peripheral nervous system is also involved in the health damage caused by lightning strikes (Kleiter et al. 2008). The pathophysiological mechanisms of the often observed neurological and psychological disorders after a lightning strike accident are unclear. The spectrum of health damage ranges from nonspecific complaints such as sensory disorders or chronic fatigue to defined disease patterns such as depression or post-traumatic stress disorder. Such long-term effects, which are reported to occur in 70–75% of all patients, can severely limit the quality of life of the accident victims (Cherington 2003; Cooray et al. 2007; Forster et al. 2013; Kleiter et al. 2007; Lederer et al. 2000; Umminger 2018; Whitcomb et al. 2002).

6.2.3.1 Classification of Injuries

In the technical literature, classifications of accidents caused by lightning strikes with damage to the central and peripheral nervous systems exist, both according to the location and the temporal occurrence of the disorders. Both orders are presented below.

6.2.3.1.1 Neurological Disorders According to Topographical Aspects

Andrews and Reisner (2017) presented a classification into eight groups according to topographical aspects of the functional disorders. They distinguished the categories:

- central syndromes,
- cerebellar syndromes,
- cranial nerve syndromes,
- autonomic syndromes,
- Disorders after spinal cord injuries,
- paralyses,
- Disorders of the peripheral nervous system and
- sensory disorders.

Central Syndromes

In the technical literature, several different cerebral syndromes have been reported after accidents caused by lightning strikes. Here, brain hemorrhages dominate in almost all variations (Caksen et al. 2004; Carrera-Izquierdo et al. 2004; Cherington 2003; Cherington et al. 1993, 1997; Guardiola et al. 2010; Knaggs 2002; Mann et al. 1983; Morgan et al. 1958; Ohashi et al. 2001; Ozgun und Castillo 1995; Stanley und Suss 1985; Steinbaum et al. 1994; Thomas et al. 1991; Wakasugi und Masui 1986). These hemorrhages are often accompanied by skull fractures. There are reports that suggest chronicity and associations with other neurological sequelae. In particular, the basal ganglia seem to be susceptible to injuries. Brain infarcts are only briefly mentioned and associated with a vascular pathomechanism (Huan-Jui et al. 2010).

Encephalopathic syndromes include confusion, amnesia, seizures, hallucinations and dysphasia, as well as the occurrence of diffuse changes in the white matter (Bryan et al. 2009; Cherington 1995; Courtman et al. 2003; Isao et al. 2005; Kleiter et al. 2007; Kruja et al. 2016; Milton et al. 1996; Paterson and Turner 1944; Poser 1994). Occasionally, findings with questionable relation to a lightning strike accident are also presented. These include, for example, glioma and brain atrophy (Cherington et al. 1994; Andrews and Reisner 2017). Electrical, thermal, mechanical and/or hypoxic effects are postulated as causative pathophysiological mechanisms (Bryan et al. 2009).

Furthermore, movement disorders are reported and the distinction between these central syndromes and peripheral movement disorders is emphasized (Cherington 2003; Morris et al. 1998; O'Brien 1995; Quinn and Maraganore 2000). In particular, Parkinsonism Parkinsonism, choreoathetosis, dystonia, myoclonus and cerebral tremor are listed under the heading of movement disorders, and basal ganglia ischemia and cerebral hypoxia are considered key mechanisms (O'Brien 1995). Jankovic and Pardo (1986) report on the electrical origin of myoclonus and also on demyelination in some of the total 18 patients in their case study.

Motor neuron disease are often reported as a syndrome with delayed onset. A similarity with amyotrophic lateral sclerosis is also mentioned. Delayed onset and slow progression seem to characterize these disorders. Some authors even report years of delay before the onset of numerous syndromes. The commonality between the generic motor neuron disease and the more specific amyotrophic lateral sclerosis is seen in both cases in the involvement of the last motor neurons in the movement pathway (Cherington 2003; Gallagher and Talbert 1991; Ghosh et al. 1995; Jafari et al. 2001; Zoccolella et al. 2008).

Cerebellar Syndromes

There are only a few reports on cerebellar syndromes (Cherington 2003; Gilbert 1994; Hey and Rieder 1983; Suri and Vijayan 1978). Cherington et al. (1993) listed 4 cases, of which 3 were regressive and in one case cerebellar atrophy followed. Gilbert (1994) presented a case study in which previous rapid and confused speech became "robotic" and postulated that this disorder was of cerebellar origin. Suri and Vijayan (1978) diagnosed cerebellar signs in a soldier who had been hit while on the phone. Cherington et al. (1995) reported on a patient with cerebellar ataxia. Another accident victim showed, in addition to cerebellar ataxia, also dysmetriaand dysdiadochokinesia (Hey and Rieder 1983). The different skull openings are considered entry points for lightning strike injuries to the cerebellum (Andrews 1992, 1995).

Cranial Nerve Syndromes

There are numerous case reports about cranial nerve lesions as a result of lightning strike accidents. The optic nerves, but also other cranial nerves, are relatively frequently affected. Thus, after lightning strikes, diplopia, mydriasis, anisocoria, Horner's syndromeand accommodation disorders have been described (Abt 1985; Baqain et al. 2004; Graber et al. 1996; Lea 1920). Norman and Younge (1999) report on a case with vision loss that responded to high-dose methylprednisolone therapy. Furthermore, case reports with facial palsyand bulbar palsy were found, which led to dysphagia (Richards 1973, Saddler and Thomas 1990; Silbergleit and Trenkner 1988). Also, patients with dysphasia were observed after lightning strike accidents (Caksen et al. 2004; Desai and Fairclough 2011; Isao et al. 2005). Furthermore, there are cases with cochleovestibular disorders, where the patients experienced dizziness, tinnitus and reduced hearing (Modayil et al. 2014; Poulsen and Knudstrup 1986).

Autonomic Syndromes

Examples of autonomic dysfunctions following a lightning strike accident include reports of patients with Sudeck's disease, causalgia, electrolyte disorders and a salt-wasting syndrome (Belsole and Smith 1990; Demun et al. 1993; Emet et al. 2010; Grubb and Karabin 2007; Hawkes and Thorpe 1992; Jost et al. 2005; Kim and Bryant 2001; Lim et al. 2001; Orbak and Kara 2010; Ozdemir et al. 2002; Rosenberg 1989; Shantha 1991; Weeramanthri et al. 1991). In at least 2 cases, a central cause for persistent arterial hypertension was postulated (Suri and Vijayan 1978; Weeramanthri et al. 1991).

Disorders Following Spinal Cord Injuries

In the case of spinal cord lesions, both immediate and delayed occurrences of amyotrophic lateral sclerosis and transverse myelopathy as well as associated demyelination processes are reported (Abhinav et al. 2007; Arévalo et al. 1999; Bariar et al. 2002; Butler and Grant 1977; Cherington 2003; Christensen et al. 1980; Clouston 1995; Davidson and Deck 1988; Deveci et al. 2001; Erkin et al. 2007; Ko et al. 2004; Koller and Orságh 1989; Lakshminarayanan et al. 2009). Furthermore, other related syndromes at the spinal level were found, for example corticospinal paresis (Johansen et al. 2008), anterior horn myelopathy (Fu et al. 2008) and dystonias (Adler and Caviness 1997; Farrell and Starr 1968; Ondo 1997). MRI findings support the diagnosis (Freemann et al. 2004).

Paralysis

Paralysis is widespread among patients affected by a lightning strike accident. All forms of paralysis can occur. There are reports of flaccid, spastic, transient, long-lasting, immediate, delayed, unilateral, and bilateral paralysis. Furthermore, there are reports of patients with lightning-induced paraplegia and tetraplegia (Baqain et al. 2004; Breugem et al. 1999; Caksen et al. 2004; Clouston 1995; Fu et al. 2008; Gathier 1988; Gouse et al. 2015; Hawkes and Thorpe 1992; Kanitkar and Roberts 1988; Ko et al. 2004; Sharma and Smith 1978; Steffen et al. 1992; Varghese et al. 1986).

A special form of paralysis after a lightning strike is keraunoparalysis (Greek: "keraunós"—lightning, "parálysi"—paralysis). In this case, the limbs become cold, pale, numb, and pulseless. Keraunoparalysis, which occurs immediately after the accident and usually heals within a few hours, is often mistaken for compartment syndrome. The cause is believed to be an electricity-induced spasm of one or more arteries responsible for supplying the affected limb (Andrews et al. 1992; Baqain et al. 2004; Breugem et al. 1999; Caksen et al. 2004; Clouston 1995; Fu et al. 2008; Gathier 1988; Gouse et al. 2015; Graber et al. 1996; Hawkes and Thorpe 1992; Kanitkar and Roberts 1988; Ko et al. 2004; Sharma and Smith 1978; Steffen et al. 1992; ten Duis et al. 1985; Varghese et al. 1986).

Disorders of the Peripheral Nervous System

After lightning strike accidents, various functional disorders of the peripheral nervous system can also occur. For example, combinations involving the median, ulnar, and radial nerves in the upper extremities have been reported (Butler and Grant 1977, Cahill et al. 2014; Clouston 1995; Engrav et al. 1990; Patnaik et al. 2015; Rosenberg 1989).

In the case of functional disorders of the peripheral nerves of the lower extremities, the sciatic and femoral nerves, as well as further peripheral branches, are predominantly affected (Butler and Grant 1977; Cahill et al. 2014; Cherington 2003; Clouston 1995;

Engrav et al. 1990; Fan et al. 2005; Mankani et al. 1994; Patnaik et al. 2015; Rosenberg 1989; Wilbourn 1995).

Cases with a Guillian-Barré-like syndrome have also been reported (Girard and Jacquot 1954; Panagiotis et al. 2008).

In connection with disorders of the peripheral nervous system, the frequently observed muscle weakness, loss of endurance, and easy fatigability are also seen (Baqain et al. 2004; Bhargava et al. 2014; Butler and Grant 1977; Clouston 1995; Courtman et al. 2003; Fu et al. 2008; Steinbaum et al. 1994). These complications are also differentially diagnosed as myopathy.

Sensory Disorders

In connection with lightning strike accidents, victims are often diagnosed with complex regional pain syndromes (Complex Regional Pain Syndrome, CRPS) (Andrews and Reisner 2017; Nield and Kamat 2004). CRPS is a collective term for conditions that affect the extremities, develop after a damaging event, and are characterized by persistent pain with disorders of the autonomic nervous system, sensitivity, and motor skills (Pschyrembel 2020). The persistent pain is often also associated with muscle weakness. Myelin sheath decay and nerve cell edema are postulated as pathomorphological mechanisms. Furthermore, it is suspected that the cause of CRPS could also lie in damage to the neuromuscular junction, which could also explain the weakness and especially the early fatigue. The sensory dysfunction may also be due to damage to the sensory nerve endings (Andrews and Reisner 2017).

6.2.3.1.2 Neurological Disorders According to the Time of Occurrence

Furthermore, Cherington 2003also presented a classification into four groups according to the time of occurrence of health impairments. The neurological and/or psychological consequences for a lightning strike victim can

- be acute and transient,
- be acute and persistent,
- be delayed, or
- occur at any time after secondary traumatic events

appear.

The *first group* of acute and transient disorders includes the immediate complications of a lightning strike accident. These consist of a temporary loss of consciousness, amnesia, aphasia, confusion, headaches, and keraunoparalysis (Muehlberger et al. 2001). Keraunoparalysis is a historical term for numerous symptoms often observed in victims of a lightning strike immediately after the accident. It consists of a spinal shock with temporary paralysis, particularly of the lower extremities, with weakness, loss of sensation, vasoconstriction, pulselessness, pallor, and arterial hypertension. A detailed description of these acute consequences of a lightning strike dates back to the French doctor Jean-Martin Charcot and the year 1887 (Jellinek 1903). Keraunoparalysis is a symptom complex characteristic of a lightning strike accident and is usually regressive in the first hours after the event (Backhaus et al. 2016; Jellinek 1903; Naik and Krishna 2018; Rahmani et al. 2015; ten Duis et al. 1985; Umminger 2018).

The *second group* includes acute consequences with long-lasting or persistent damage. This primarily includes posthypoxic encephalopathy, which has a poor prognosis and either leads to death after a latency period or to extensive cognitive deficits in the survivor. In addition to this brain damage, intracerebral hemorrhages, particularly in the area of the basal ganglia and brainstem, cerebralinfarcts, myelopathies, and nonspecific atrophies can also lead to permanent health damage (Backhaus et al. 2016; Umminger 2018).

The *third group* includes the delayed and progressively occurring complications of a lightning strike accident. These include motor neuron diseases, movement disorders, neuropathies, seizure disorders, chronic headaches, and other consequences. The mentioned complications of a lightning strike can occur days, weeks, months, or years after the event, with the pathophysiological correlations with the lightning strike not yet clarified (Backhaus et al. 2016; Reisner 2013; Umminger 2018).

The *fourth group* includes all secondary traumatic consequences of a lightning strike, which can occur both immediately and after a latency period. These include all neurological and psychological complications, for example, caused by fall events with consecutive traumatic subdural, epidural, or subarachnoid hemorrhages (Backhaus et al. 2016).

Case Study

A 51-year-old woman suffered an accident at night in her home in India when a lightning strike hit the house during a thunderstorm. The outer wall of the house subsequently showed a deep crack, and shards of a shattered window were scattered in the living room. The injured woman was taken to a clinic the same night. Upon admission, she exhibited pronounced muscle weakness on the right side of her body, lack of sensation in the extremities and the right half of her face, as well as dizziness. Her arms and legs felt cold. Vital functions were inconspicuous. The patient showed no external injuries. A diagnosis of keraunoparalysis was made and infusion therapy with 0.9% saline solution in conjunction with parenteral administration of betamethasone and ranitidine was initiated. A significant regression of the complaints occurred within 4 hours. The motor weakness completely disappeared, the loss of sensation only partially. Due to the dizziness, the patient vomited twice. The lightning strike victim was discharged from the clinic after 2 days. At a follow-up examination after a week, she still had minimal dizziness and discrete sensory disturbances in the extremities (Naik and Krishna 2018). ◄

6.2.3.2 Diagnosis

Clinical Examinations

Even in the early phase of treating a lightning strike victim, the patient may exhibit non-obvious damage to organs or organ systems. Therefore, a thorough inventory of accident-related functional restrictions is necessary, not only for forensic reasons. If there is suspicion of neurological or psychological deficits, the consultation of a relevant consulting physician is obligatory. Early psychological care is explicitly recommended if needed (Backhaus et al. 2016; Baxter 1970; Chico et al. 1999; Zasler 1996).

In clinical-neurological examinations, different findings can occur depending on the course of the current flow. In the acute phase, keraunoparalysis is often diagnosed. This often involves a loss of muscle tone with paresis and a vasospasm syndrome with the clinical finding of pulselessness and cooling of the extremities. Furthermore, complex regional pain syndromes can occur in the acute phase (ten Duis et al. 1985). These complications, which are potentially reversible, are considered to be due to a central nervous autonomic disorder (Jost et al. 2005). This cause, in addition to a direct influence of the electric current on the cardiac conduction system, is also discussed as a trigger for the ventricular fibrillation often observed in the acute phase (Backhaus et al. 2016).

Furthermore, almost all types of peripheral and/or central neurological disorders can be observed. Special attention should be paid to complications in anesthetized patients, as these may be overlooked. For example, conscious accident victims report lightning-induced glare effects that can lead to the development of an electric cataract or other eye damage. Therefore, clinical examinations by doctors of different specialties are recommended for patients with impaired consciousness.

Imaging

The computed tomography (CT scan, CT) has its dominant role in the acute diagnosis of patients who have suffered a lightning strike. It serves, for example, for the rapid diagnosis of fractures or intracranial injuries and should be performed in all patients with consciousness disorders or other neurological deficits. However, an unremarkable CT can lead to a performed magnetic resonance imaging (MRI) revealing various pathological findings. Case reports include subarachnoid hemorrhages, bithalamic hemorrhages, white matter lesions, and myelon damage (Backhaus et al. 2016; Johansen et al. 2008; Ozgun and Castillo 1995). In addition, imaging diagnostics make a relevant contribution to excluding competing causes of the detected neurological lesions in patients.

Neurophysiological Examination Methods

In victims of a lightning strike who develop a chronic pain syndrome or suffer from sensitive sensations with hypo- or paresthesias, neurophysiological examination methods can provide evidence of lesions of sensitive peripheral nerve fibers. In particular, quantitative sensory testing (QST) and the recording of the sympathetic skin response (SSR) are relevant. From a pathophysiological point of view, the development of polyneuropathy due to lesions of the thinly myelinated A-delta fibers and the unmyelinated C-fibers is discussed (Hawkes and Thorpe 1992; Nebuchennykh et al. 2009). In these patients, no pathological findings are often found with other neurophysiological methods, such as electromyography (EMG) and electroneurography (ENG).

The extremely high current strengths that occur during a lightning strike can lead to damage to thickly myelinated nerve fibers. These axonal lesions can be detected with EMG and ENG (Davidson and Deck 1988; Wilbourn 1995).

Electroencephalography

There are no systematic studies in the literature on the electroencephalographic diagnosis after lightning strike injuries in humans. After direct lightning strikes to the head, both generalized and focal pathological changes in the Electroencephalogram (EEG) have been described (Kruse 1966). Furthermore, generalized encephalopathic changes without image morphological correlate have been documented over a period of several months after a lightning strike accident (Kleiter et al. 2007). In most cases, however, EEG changes typically correspond with the lightning-induced morphological findings on the skin of the head (Kruse 1966). Occasionally, focal findings independent of the primary lesion, without correlation in an MRI of the head, are described. In one case report, a focal finding was still detectable in follow-up examinations 18 months later (Kleiter et al. 2007).

There are currently no studies on EEG changes that are attributable to lightning-induced hypoxic brain damage or other secondary consequences. In an overall view, EEG diagnostics are considered useful in the presence of corresponding symptoms, as focal findings that do not have image morphological correlates can be uncovered as indications of an accident-related symptomatic epilepsy (Backhaus et al. 2016).

Examinations Relevant to the Diagnosis of Lightning-Induced Neurological Damage

- Clinical examination
- Imaging (CT, MRI)
- Neurophysiological examination methods (QST, SSR, EMG, ENG)
- EEG

6.2.3.3 Neuropsychological Consequences

The effects of electric current on the human body are never limited to the areas of direct contact. Touching electrical power sources can lead to a significant strain on the particularly conductive nerve pathways, so that contact with any part of the body can also cause cerebral lesions (Duff and McCaffrey 2001). The literature shows that exposure of the nervous system to electric current can result in significant impairment of performance and coordinated activation of cognitive processes (Pliskin et al. 1998; Reisner 2006; Silversides 1964). These changes were observed in patients who had contact with the electric current outside the head region. The observed performance deficits were not only limited to the acute phase. In a functional MRI study, Ramati et al. (2009) described that the coordination of activation patterns in patients after an electrical trauma differed significantly from the patterns of healthy control subjects. These differences were reflected in a significantly weaker performance of memory and attention in the accident victims. Even with still standard performances of the patients, a comparison with the general performance level can be used to check whether the differences significantly deviate from the general level and should be classified as newly acquired or as pre-existing variance. The general performance level is measured with intelligence tests and supplementary methods for visuoperception and attention. The variance of performance impairments after lightning strike accidents shows a considerable range. These deficits can reach such a degree of severity that the individual's insight into the accident-related performance losses is impaired. This can even go so far that these impairments can no longer be perceived.

It is not uncommon for accident victims to be told by medical colleagues who do not represent the specialties of neurology, psychiatry or ophthalmology that they have had "luck in misfortune" and are now recovered after their therapy. If they subsequently become overwhelmed when confronted with everyday life and the associated professional and domestic demands, this is often seen as post-traumatic stress disorder. It is sometimes overlooked that some of the disorders that have occurred are due to neuronal damage (Backhaus et al. 2016).

Common Neuropsychological Consequences of a Lightning Accident

- Memory impairment
- Cognitive disorders
- Attention deficits

6.2.3.4 Psychiatric Consequences

There are no systematic studies in the literature about psychiatric diseases that have occurred as a result of lightning strike accidents. However, there are numerous case reports about a delayed onset of symptoms in the sense of a post-traumatic stress disorder as well as specific or generalized anxiety disorders. In this context, a lack of professional knowledge and understanding by treating doctors, family members, friends and/or colleagues can act as an intensifying factor. This experience, as well as the realization of a possible neuropsychic performance reduction, can lead to social withdrawal tendencies as well as family and professional problems. In this context, patients are also reported who have developed symptoms of a manifest depressionas a result of the accident (Reisner 2006).

A defined external event with extraordinary psychological stress is the indispensable prerequisite for the development of a post-traumatic stress disorder (Blanchard et al. 1996; Frommberger et al. 2014). The occurrence of this health damage is also described after accidents caused by lightning strikes (Backhaus et al. 2016; Zack et al. 2010). In contrast to victims of rape, who develop an acute stress reaction in more than 90% and a post-traumatic stress disorder in about 50% of cases, victims of lightning strikes or other natural disasters show significantly lower frequencies (Kessler et al. 1995; Resnick et al. 2007). In addition to the trauma, the diagnosis also includes re-experiencing, avoidance behavior, hyperarousal, and psychosocial impairments. The mentioned disorders must persist for more than a month (Frommberger et al. 2014). The acute stress reaction is to be distinguished from the post-traumatic stress disorder in the phase immediately after the accident. In this case, after an initial feeling of "numbness", usually changing symptoms such as despair, anger, hyperactivity or disorientation occur, which usually subside within hours to days. Since a post-traumatic stress disorder is relatively well treatable, the symptoms should be treated without delay in case of a suspicion of such a disorder. Most trauma therapies are carried out on an outpatient basis. Only when the intensity, severity, and complexity of the symptoms exceed the outpatient possibilities, inpatient therapy in a specialized clinic should be considered. The treatment of patients with a post-traumatic stress disorder consists of psychotherapies and the administration of psychotropic drugs (Frommberger et al. 2014).

After the symptoms have subsided, a further neuropsychological examination can more precisely capture a neuronally caused performance reduction (Backhaus et al. 2016).

Possible Psychiatric Consequences of a Lightning Strike Accident

- Acute Stress Reaction
- Post-Traumatic Stress Disorder
- Depression
- Anxiety Disorder

6.2.3.5 Rehabilitation

In rehabilitation, a distinction must be made between acute trauma consequences and long-term sequelae. The rehabilitation of severely injured lightning strike victims does not differ from the measures for patients who have a different cause for their health damage (Backhaus et al. 2016; Lammertse 2005). A large period of time should be considered when planning rehabilitation treatments. The rehabilitation process after a severe lightning strike accident can extend over months, years, or even a lifetime (Dobkin 2003, Katz et al. 2004; Pliskin et al. 1998). The rehabilitation treatment must always be oriented towards the dominant injury pattern. The goal of all rehabilitative measures is to minimize the physical, psychological, and neuropsychological consequences of a lightning strike injury. A focus of the treatment is to enable the patient to lead as independent a life as possible (Greenberger and Padesky 2015; Heilbronner and Pliskin 1999; Umminger 2018).

Long-term effects are mostly characterized by clinically difficult to detect symptoms such as neurocognitive performance impairments and/or psychological impairments. Personality changes and disorders of attention, concentration, and sleep or abnormal daytime sleepiness are often the reason for disability and social withdrawal. In this context, neuropathic symptoms and chronic pain syndromes also play a role. Pain that occurs, for example, after brain injuries is often central pain. Here, physiotherapies and centrally acting analgesics are particularly indicated (Bowsher 1995; Martinelli et al. 2004).

For the treating doctors, diagnosing the symptoms and for the patients, acknowledging the health damages as a result of the accident can sometimes be a hurdle. Especially with early detection of deficits and targeted therapy coordinated with them, the prognosis can be good. Parallel to the neurophysiological rehabilitation measures, consistent diagnostics and initiation of therapy must be carried out early if there are indications of emerging psychological disorders. Behavioral and drug treatments are in the foreground (Dobkin 2003; Kessler 2000; Primeau et al. 1995; Primeau 2005; Yarnell 2005).

Because the long-term sequelae are underdiagnosed, in many cases it is indicated for patients with lightning strike injuries to present in a specialized clinic to initiate targeted diagnostics (Backhaus et al. 2016; Davis et al. 2014). From a neurological point of view, an early presentation of apparently inconspicuous patients is recommended in order to, for example, record a neurocognitive baseline status and to be able to delineate subsequent impairments in the course. This approach is of considerable relevance for expert opinion, as the sequelae of a lightning strike can lead to a reduction in earning capacity of up to 100% for a victim (Frommberger et al. 2013). Patients should also be informed that they should immediately report to the responsible professional association in the event of an occupational or commuting accident.

Key Features of Rehabilitation Treatment for Patients with Persistent Complications After a Lightning Strike Accident

- Depending on the severity of the injuries, there are different treatment successes.
- Long-term effects also require long rehabilitation processes.
- Preferred treatments include psychotherapies, physiotherapies, occupational therapies and pain therapies.
- The goals are to minimize the consequences and to lead as independent a life as possible.

6.2.4 Audiovestibular System

While injuries to the ear due to accidents involving technical electricity are rare, they occur in more than half of all cases involving lightning strikes (Makin 2023, Tribble et al. 1985). Individuals struck by lightning can exhibit a variety of different otological damages. The most common injuries in the field of otolaryngology (ENT) are undoubtedly the tympanic membrane ruptures that can be detected immediately after the barotrauma has occurred. But also hearing impairments, tinnitus, and balance disorders are often reported after such events. All other lightning-related health damages in the ENT area are rather rare (Table 6.5).

6.2.4.1 Tympanic Membrane Rupture

In a study on fatal accidents caused by lightning strikes, Wetli (1996) found tympanic membrane ruptures in 17 out of 21 (81%) victims, which occurred unilaterally in 10 cases and bilaterally in 7 cases. In a selected patient group from the Department of Otorhinolaryngology at the University of Split (Croatia), 12 out of 18 (66.6%) victims of a lightning strike had a unilateral or bilateral tympanic membrane rupture. Upon admission to the clinic, all 12 patients simultaneously complained of severe pain, tinnitus, and hearing loss (Glunic et al. 2001).

Case Study

A 24-year-old woman in Mecklenburg-Western Pomerania (Germany) was thrown to the ground, unconscious, and subsequently without spontaneous breathing due to a direct lightning strike. After successful intensive medical treatment and termination of analgesia, the patient complained on the 3rd day after the accident of watery ear

Table 6.5 Possible audiovestibular consequences of a lightning strike. (Own illustration)

Injury/Symptom	Authors
Tympanic membrane rupture	Blumenthal 2021; Bozan et al. 2016; Gluncic et al. 2001; Junkins et al. 1999; Kleiter et al. 2007
Hearing loss	Angerer et al. 2009; Junkins et al. 1999; Just et al. 2002; Kubilius and Rimdeika 2012
Tinnitus	Angerer et al. 2009; Epperly and Stewart 1989; Jones et al. 1991; Kubilius and Rimdeika 2012
Vertigo	Just et al. 2002; Kilic et al. 2017; Youngs et al. 1988
Otalgia	Angerer et al. 2009
Dislocation of the ossicles	Offiah et al. 2007
Oval window fistulas	Jones et al. 1991

secretion, hearing loss, and tinnitus on the left side, as well as temporary dizziness. The patient was then transferred to an ENT clinic. The initial findings there showed thermal injuries to the neck and left foot, as well as otoscopically a two-quadrant defect of the left tympanic membrane, thermal damage to the bony ear canal near the tympanic membrane, and a reddened mucous membrane of the tympanic cavity. The right tympanic membrane was unremarkable. The tone audiogram showed a combined hearing loss on the left with an inner ear component in all frequencies between 30 and 40 dB with normal hearing on the right. The stapedius reflex on the left had disappeared. After an infusion therapy containing mannitol, administration of an antibiotic, and ear care, there was an increase in the hearing curve on the left, a regression of the ear secretion, and healing of the burns on the ear. After a recovery process of 3.5 months, the left tympanic membrane showed no pathological findings anymore (Just et al. 2002). ◀

Gordon et al. (1995) provide the following recommendations for the management and therapy of affected patients based on their experience in treating 4 accident victims in Florida (USA), in combination with the specialist literature:

- As with any other traumatic perforation, the external ear canal should be cleaned and the inverted edges of the tympanic membrane should be everted.
- Thorough microscopic examinations should be carried out to rule out the development of a cholesteatoma.
- If there is no specific indication for early surgical intervention, it is advisable to wait at least a few months due to the self-healing tendency of the tympanic membrane before a tympanoplasty is performed.
- If a tympanoplasty is performed, the surgeon should be aware of potential problems that may arise during postoperative healing.

In the German-language specialist literature, a guideline of the German Society for General Medicine and Family Medicine (2014), which is currently being revised, recommends that follow-up examinations of patients should be carried out until the complete closure of the lesion in the case of a simple, small tear in the tympanic membrane. Due to the risk of otitis media, no ear irrigations or ear drops should be used. Depending on the symptoms, antibiotic therapy may be indicated. In the case of larger ruptures, there is a tendency for the edges of the tympanic membrane to roll in. In these cases, a rapid adaptation of the wound edges should be carried out by an ENT specialist using an otoscope. Due to the lack of review articles on traumatically caused tympanic membrane ruptures, the recommendations mentioned are based on expert opinions and textbook knowledge.

Characteristic Clinical Audiovestibular Symptoms and Findings

- More than half of all surviving victims of a lightning strike show audiovestibular symptoms and/or findings.
- Tympanic membrane ruptures are most common and can occur unilaterally or bilaterally. They have a good tendency to self-heal.
- Occurring hearing impairments due to conductive hearing loss mostly have a good prognosis.
- Vertigo is the most common vestibular symptom and rapidly regressive.
- Inner ear damages are rare, but can lead to hearing loss.

6.2.5 Visual System

At the moment of a lightning strike accident, both the electric current flowing through the head and the strong radiation emanating from the plasma channel can cause a number of medical problems in the eye. Numerous ocular complications develop over a long period of time, so a longer monitoring of survivors of a lightning strike is required (Andrews et al. 1992; Cooray et al. 2007; Espaillat et al. 1999; Norman et al. 2001).

6.2.5.1 Cataract

Cataract or grey star is the most common long-term injury observed after accidents caused by lightning strikes (Cataracta electrica) (Tribble et al. 1985). The first lightning-induced cataract was documented more than 300 years ago in France (St Yves 1722). A grey star is the clouding of the eye lens, which impairs vision. A cataract occurs more frequently bilaterally than unilaterally after a lightning strike (Tribble et al. 1985).

After a lightning strike injury, two types of cataract are distinguished. The first type is due to a concussion of the head, which leads to slight tears in the lens capsule. This traumatic cataract occurs shortly after the event (Tribble et al. 1985). The other type is caused by the various radiations associated with a lightning strike. The lens is mainly composed of water and proteins. If these proteins denature, for example, due to high temperatures and/or ultraviolet (UV) radiation, it clouds the lens and reduces the light that reaches the retina. In fact, the lightning channel is a very strong source of UV, X-ray, and gamma radiation (Cooray et al. 2007; Dwyer et al. 2003). A cataract caused by radiation can sometimes only occur after a considerable latency period, which can also be years (Table 6.6) (Elsom 2000; Tribble et al. 1985).

According to Duke-Elder and McFaul (1972), after an accident caused by high-voltage electricity, anterior subcapsular changes are predominantly observed, while a lightning strike causes cloudiness in both the anterior and posterior capsule. Noel et al. (1980) noticed fine lines in the posterior subcapsular areas 7 weeks after a lightning strike accident. In the 14th week after the event, a dense posterior subcapsular cloudiness was recognizable without anterior subcapsular changes. As a general rule, lens cloudi-

Table 6.6 Temporal occurrence of a cataract after a lightning strike. (Own illustration)

Age (years)	Gender	Latency	Authors
n. s.	n. s.	3 months	Kubilius and Rimdeika 2012
9	m	5 months	Dinakaran et al. 1998
19	m	6 months	Hawkes and Thorpe 1992
57	f	>40 years	Venkateswaran and Galor 2018

m male, f female, n. s. not specified

ness follows a lightning strike faster than after an accident caused by high-voltage electricity. Cataracts can also occur years after the lightning strike accident.

The occurrence of a cataract has been observed not only in outdoor lightning strikes, but also in indoor accidents associated with the use of corded telephones (Dinakaran et al. 1998). In addition to cataracts, there are numerous other effects of lightning strikes on the human eye region, the most important of which are described below.

6.2.5.2 Retinal Damage

The retina is the sensory receiving surface of the eye, evolutionarily a part of the brain, and lines the inside of the eye. The visual information received there is transmitted to the brain via the optic nerve. The central region of the retina, which contains a high density of photoreceptors, is referred to as the macula. The macula provides the sharp, central vision we need to see the smallest details. Lightning strikes can cause damage to the macula, causing acute blurred and distorted central vision (Cooray et al. 2007). Such an injury is referred to as a macular hole (Rao et al. 2009). The lightning injury can cause the retina to warp or shift from its normal position. Such damages are referred to as retinal detachment ("ablatio retinae"). In addition to retinal detachment, lightning strikes can cause folds in the retinal tissue in one or more sections of the retina. These damages cause small blind spots and are also called "retinal folds" (Cooray et al. 2007; Espaillat et al. 1999).

Retinoschisis, chorioretinal atrophy, macular edema, maculopathy, hemorrhages, pigment disorders, and the appearance of fibrous membranes have also been described on the retina following lightning strike accidents (Dhillon and Gupta 2015; Harris et al. 2019; Kubilius and Rimdeika 2012; Moore 1956; Noel et al. 1980; Pradhan et al. 2020; Rao et al. 2009; Tribble et al. 1985).

6.2.5.3 Inflammations

After a lightning strike accident, there can also be local inflammations of the eye. Patients with conjunctivitis, keratitis, iritis, iridocyclitisand uveitis have been particularly described (Hawkes and Thorpe 1992; Iranyi et al. 1962; Kubilius and Rimdeika 2012; Pradhan et al. 2020; Rao et al. 2009; Stütz et al. 2006).

Lea (1920) reports an accident followed by conjunctivitis in combination with a mild ciliary muscle paresis, accommodation disorders and photophobia.

Inflammations of the cornea can manifest either through a transient focal or a severe interstitial keratitis with ulceration or perforation (Taussig 1968; Tribble et al. 1985; Volinsky et al. 1994).

For iridocyclitis, both a mild short-term and a severe chronic course are described (Tribble et al. 1985).

In the case of uveitis, there can be extreme light sensitivity (photophobia) (Cooray et al. 2007).

6.2.5.4 Further Damages

After a lightning strike accident, in addition to cataracts, retinal lesions, and inflammations, there can be numerous other injuries and long-term effects on the human visual organ.

Hanson and McIlwraith (1973) report an event with bilateral blindness, which was attributed to atrophy of the optic nerves. In another accident, a complete loss of vision, which lasted only 20 minutes, was documented (Taussig 1968). Norman and Younge (1999) describe a patient who, after a lightning strike, had no light perception and unresponsive pupils with unremarkable fundus findings on both sides and regained full vision in both eyes after intravenous methylprednisolone therapy. Whether the therapy was causally responsible for the recovery remained open.

During a lightning strike, strong ultraviolet and high-energy radiation can penetrate the eye and cause various injuries. The cornea is a layer of protective and light-transmitting tissue that covers the iris in the front part of the eyeball. Indeed, it is the cornea that suffers the main part of the damage when the eyes are exposed to high-energy radiation. This can result in corneal burns, swelling edema, corneal opacities, ulcers, and punctate keratitis. Changes or complete loss of vision can occur. Lightning can also lead to double vision (diplopia), which is due to damage to the eye muscles or their nerve supply. The ability to read, walk, and perform general activities is suddenly impaired. In one case, a young girl experienced a reversal of the optical image after a lightning strike, so she perceived the outside world upside down for some time.

A lightning strike injury can cause the vitreous body to detach from the retina. In addition, a lightning strike can also cause bleeding into the vitreous body (Cooray et al. 2007).

Furthermore, burns of the conjunctiva and cornea have been described, which can also be associated with ulcers and necrosis (Iranyi et al. 1962; Raule 1986; Tribble et al. 1985).

As a late consequence of a lightning strike, scars and/or atrophies can occur in different regions of the eye (Harris et al. 2019). After a direct hit to the head, Wankhede and Sariya (2013) found significant bleeding of the sclera.

Case Study

A 16-year-old girl was injured by a lightning strike in India in April 2008 while she was sleeping on the floor of her house at night. In this accident, a relative who was about 2 m away from her was killed.

Although she had noticed blurred vision in her right eye and hearing loss in her right ear immediately after the event, she only presented to an ophthalmologist two months later due to a sudden painless deterioration in vision.

On examination in an eye clinic, a significant reduction in visual acuity was found on the right. The intraocular pressure was 12 and 10 mmHg, respectively. The examinations revealed a relative afferent pupillary defect of the right eye and bilateral subcapsular cataract. The fundus examination showed bilateral macular holes and several areas of hyperpigmentation of the retinal pigment epithelium in the periphery of both eyes. Fluorescein angiography showed increased choroidal transmission with early fluorescence and late fading in the foveal region and retinal pigment epithelium speckling in the periphery of the eyes. The clinical examinations showed no abnormal findings in pulse, blood pressure, and kidney function. The skin and eyelids showed no burns. At a follow-up examination 3 months after the accident, the young woman was found to have anterior uveitis of the right eye and was treated with topical steroids and cycloplegics. No further information is available on the course of the disease (Rao et al. 2009). ◀

6.2.5.5 Therapy and Outcome

The therapy for ocular complications of a lightning strike accident is carried out according to existing standards and guidelines, depending on the diagnosis. In particular, persistent complaints and late effects are often reported with eye injuries. Thus, Pradhan et al. (2020) documented no improvement in 4 out of 7 disease courses within weeks to months.

Characteristics of Eye Injuries After Lightning Strike

- Eye injuries often occur after lightning strike accidents.
- In events involving the eyes, lens opacities and retinal lesions dominate.
- Overall, there is a wide variety of possible ocular injuries and late effects for this type of accident. Persistent complaints are not uncommon.
- Long-term follow-up is necessary for many patients.

6.2.6 Respiratory Tract

After a lightning strike accident with a direct hit or a side flash, an immediate respiratory arrest is often reported. The cause is seen in an acute damage to the central nervous system, especially the respiratory center (Cooper 1980; Cooper et al. 2017; Cwinn and Cantrill 1985). Furthermore, tachypnea can sometimes be observed in the first hours and days after the accident, which can have different causes (Oflu et al. 2021; Sener et al. 2019). In addition to these functional disorders of pulmonary respiration, pulmonary injuries also occur in such events, where pathomorphological findings can be determined. Compared to other organs and organ systems, the frequency of injuries to the respiratory tract in connection with lightning strikes is rather rare. Thus, Wetli (1996), who evaluated a total of 43 autopsy cases, did not observe a lung finding related to the accident in any case. Nevertheless, there are occasional case reports in the literature about lightning-induced lung injuries (Table 6.7). Pulmonary hemorrhages are relatively frequently mentioned (Kilbas et al. 2008; Krauland 1951; Murty 2009; Oflu et al. 2021; Ohashi et al. 2001; Soltermann et al. 1991). The causes of such hemorrhages are considered to be ruptures of the alveolar walls due to the sustained barotrauma and/or contusions due to falls after the victims were thrown away from the accident site. Other rare consequences of a lightning strike accident can include burns of the larynx, a skin and soft tissue emphysema, hemothorax, pneumomediastinum, pleural effusion or aspiration pneumonia (Blumenthal and Saayman 2017; Halldorsson and Couch 2004; McCrady-Kahn and Kahn 1981; Möhle et al. 2015; Moulson 1984; Pizzi et al. 2023; Sener et al. 2019; van Waes et al. 2014). The pneumonia caused by the aspiration of vomit in the early phase after the lightning strike is also considered a consequence of central nervous

Table 6.7 Pathological findings in the respiratory tract as a result of a lightning strike accident. (Own representation)

Age (Years)	Gender	Finding	Further Consequences of Lightning Strike	Outcome	Authors
8	m	Hemothorax	Yes	Survived	van Waes et al. 2014
10	m	Aspiration Pneumonia	Yes	Deceased	McCrady-Kahn and Kahn 1981
15	m	Pulmonary Hemorrhage	Yes	Survived	Oflu et al. 2021
16	f	Pulmonary Hemorrhage	Yes	Deceased	Krauland 1951
18	m	Subcutaneous Emphysema	No	Survived	Moulson 1984
19	m	Pleural Effusions	Yes	Survived	Sener et al. 2019
20	m	Pulmonary Hemorrhage	Yes	Deceased	Ohashi et al. 2001
22	m	Pulmonary Hemorrhage	Yes	Deceased	Kilbas et al. 2008
28	m	Pneumomediastinum	No	Survived	Halldorsson and Couch 2004
35	m	Aspiration pneumonia	Yes	Deceased	Möhle et al. 2015
41	f	Pneumomediastinum	Yes	Deceased	Blumenthal and Saayman 2017
68	m	Pulmonary hemorrhage	Yes	Survived	Soltermann et al. 1991
n. s.	m	Pulmonary hemorrhage	Yes	Deceased	Murty 2009

m male, f female, n. s. not specified

system damage. The chest pain dependent on breathing and/or pulmonary edema that occur shortly after an accident are usually associated with simultaneous injury to the heart and subsequent cardiac dysfunction (see Sect. 6.2.2).

Case Study

A 15-year-old boy was with his parents and sister in an open vehicle in a field in Turkey during a thunderstorm when he was thrown about 3 m away simultaneously with a loud noise. During the clinical examination in the emergency room, he was conscious and could remember the event. The boy showed a slight tachycardia with normal respiratory rate and normotonia. The skin on the groin, ankle, dorsum of the foot, and sole of the foot on the right side showed second-degree burns. Laboratory and X-ray examinations carried out on the day of admission initially revealed no pathological findings. On the 4th day after the accident, the boy developed slight shortness of breath. A repeat chest X-ray showed a heterogeneous shadowing of the lower zone of the left lung and a blunting of the left sinus phrenicocostalis. A contrast-enhanced CT of the thorax showed ground-glass opacities in the left lower lobe of the lung. The findings were consistent with a lung contusion and alveolar bleeding. After oxygen therapy via a face mask, the shortness of breath improved on the 6th day after the accident. A chest X-ray control showed that the pulmonary hemorrhage had spontaneously resorbed. The boy was discharged from the clinic on the 9th day after the accident without any complaints. A follow-up examination 3 months later was unremarkable (Oflu et al. 2021). ◄

Therapy and Outcome

The therapy for pulmonary complications of a lightning strike accident is diagnosis-dependent according to current standards and guidelines. In the professional literature, there is no accident victim with a lethal course in which the injuries to the respiratory tract alone would have led to death. However, accident-related consequences, such as aspiration pneumonia or pulmonary hemorrhages, were identified, which had contributed to the cause of death in lethal accidents.

Characteristics of Symptoms and Complications of the Respiratory Tract after Lightning Strike

- The often observed immediate apnea in severe lightning strike accidents is a functional disorder and is most likely due to a central nervous system damage in the area of the medulla oblongata.
- Apnea is the critical factor for the outcome. Therefore, artificial ventilation must be continued after ROSC (see Sect. 6.2.2).

- Pathomorphologically detectable consequences of a lightning strike for the respiratory tract can include pulmonary hemorrhages, pneumonia due to aspiration of vomit, cases with pneumomediastinum, pleural effusions, as well as skin and/or soft tissue emphysema.
- All mentioned complications are rare.

6.2.7 Musculoskeletal System

An accident caused by a lightning strike can damage the musculoskeletal system in various ways. Victims of lightning strikes may have traumatic bone fractures, joint dislocations, or effects on the skeletal muscles.

6.2.7.1 Bone Fractures

During a lightning strike, the temperature of the lightning channel can rise to about 30,000 °C within a fraction of a second. This rapid heating leads to an explosive expansion of the heated air in the immediate vicinity of the lightning channel. The pressure wave associated with the lightning can not only damage eyes and ears, but also other internal organs (Graber et al. 1996). In addition, the pressure wave can throw the victim away, often leading to traumatic injuries (Blumenthal et al. 2012; Murty 2009; Oflu et al. 2021). A person can also be injured by flying parts of a struck object, such as a tree. Indeed, the doctor treating a victim of a lightning strike must always keep in mind the possibly associated blunt trauma (Cooray et al. 2007; Danielson et al. 2000; Matthews and Fahey 1997; Oflu et al. 2021). However, bone fractures have also been observed after a direct hit to the head (Tibesar et al. 2000). Bone fractures are most likely to occur in the area of the skull and extremities (Table 6.8).

Table 6.8 Bone fractures following a lightning strike accident. (Own illustration)

Age (Years)	Gender	Location	Authors
17	m	Femur	Netchiporouk et al. 2015
37	m	Mandible	Offiah et al. 2007
41	f	Metacarpal	Kannan et al. 2004
44	m	Temporal bone	Ohashi et al. 2001
n. s.	f	Tibia, Fibula, Midfoot	Hegner 1917
n. s.	m	Skull, Humerus	Skan 1949
n. s.	m	Skull	Tibesar et al. 2000

m male, f female, n. s. not specified

Case Study

A 41-year-old right-handed graphic designer suffered a severe injury to her right hand when lightning struck her house in England while she was operating a light switch at that moment. The lightning strike caused a massive soft tissue injury with skin loss over the thumb pad. On clinical examination, the right thumb was ischemic and numb. The index finger had reduced sensitivity and the ring finger suffered a circumferential deep burn. The X-ray examination showed a Bennet dislocation fracture of the first metacarpal in combination with a scapho-trapezio-trapezoidal dislocation. In the subsequent operation, the thenar muscles, the adductor pollicis muscle, and the first dorsal and palmar interosseous muscles could not be preserved. The lumbricales muscle of the index finger was partially torn and of questionable preservability. The palmar aponeurosis showed a split. A radical debridement was performed. The metacarpal fracture was fixed with a volar T-plate and the scapho-trapezio-trapezoidal dislocation was reduced and held with two Kirschner wires. The thumb was revascularized with a vein graft and an end-to-side anastomosis was performed with the radial artery. Nerve grafts were taken from the lateral cutaneous nerve of the forearm to reconstruct the finger nerves of the thumb and index finger. The thumb was fixed in abduction by wiring the first and second metacarpal bones together. Furthermore, a fasciotomy and split skin grafting of the ring finger were performed. The soft tissue coverage of the thumb pad was done with a combined groin and lower abdominal flap. Postoperatively, early physiotherapy was started.

At the review 12 months later, the patient had developed an intrinsic minus claw deformity of the thumb and index finger. The index finger deformity was actively and passively correctable. The thumb had a fixed flexion deformity at the interphalangeal joint. The first ray was held in an adducted position and the thumb was supinated. These problems affected the patient in daily life and prevented her from working as a graphic designer.

To improve thumb function, a flexor pollicis longus adduction opponensplasty was performed by relocating the muscle around the ulnar edge of the palmar aponeurosis. The interphalangeal joint of the thumb was fused with percutaneous Kirschner wires. A volar plate capsulodesis was performed to correct the claw deformity of the index finger. After reconstruction, the patient had improved functionality of the thumb and index finger. Although the consequences of the lightning strike had changed her grip, she was able to return to her profession as a graphic designer (Kannan et al. 2004). ◀

6.2.7.2 Damage to the Skeletal Muscles

In comparison to accidents caused by technical high voltage, injuries to the skeletal muscles after a lightning strike are less frequently observed (Cooper et al. 2017). Because lightning-related damage to the skeletal muscles can occur without noticeable skin lesions, they are sometimes overlooked (Kirchmair and Dienstl 1982; Kobernick 1982; Zack et al. 1997). The presence of significant injuries to the skeletal muscles often only becomes apparent through the results of laboratory tests in the form of increased myoglobin concentrations in serum and urine (Amy et al. 1985; Epperly and Stewart 1989; Zack et al. 1997). After a lightning accident, rhabdomyolysis is observed, which can lead to acute tubular necrosis of the toxic type and in isolated cases also to acute renal failure (see Sect. 6.2.8) (Blumenthal 2021, Hawkes and Thorpe 1992; Jitsuiki et al. 2020; Khan 2009; Okafur 2005; Sleihwah et al. 2018; Whitcomb et al. 2002; Zack et al. 2013). Occurring compartment syndromes are treated by fasciotomies (Cooper et al. 2017). In the case of a 27-year-old man who had received a side flash while standing in a tent and survived the accident for 5 days, the extensively cooked left chest muscles were only discovered at autopsy with intact skin (Zack et al. 1997). After lightning strikes, myopathies, muscle pain, and cases with a reduction in muscle strength are also described (Cherington 1995; Duppel et al. 2009; Iranyi et al. 1962; O'Keefe Gatewood and Zane 2004; Peters 1983; Ritenour et al. 2008).

Therapy and Outcome

In the treatment of bone fractures and damage to the skeletal muscles after lightning accidents, there are no peculiarities compared to other traumatic causes of such injuries. Therefore, therapy and follow-up care are carried out according to current standards and guidelines. The healing of bone fractures is usually uncomplicated. In patients with significant injuries to the skeletal muscles, lethal courses are also described, often with severe combined injuries (Whitcomb et al. 2002; Zack et al. 1997, 2013).

Characteristics of Injuries to the Musculoskeletal System After Lightning Strike

- In accidents caused by lightning strikes, the musculoskeletal system is often affected.
- Bone fractures usually occur in connection with the pressure wave accompanying a lightning strike and preferentially affect the skull and extremities.
- A lightning accident can be associated with missing external and severe internal injuries.
- In the case of damage to the skeletal muscles, rhabdomyolysis, compartment syndrome, and necrosis due to cooking are in the foreground.

6.2.8 Kidneys

After a lightning strike accident, extensive damage to the skeletal muscles can occur due to rhabdomyolysis, which is primarily reflected in significantly increased serum concentrations of creatinine, creatine kinase (CK) and potassium (Brumback et al. 1995; Pschyrembel 2020). A direct injury to the skeletal muscles or a changed metabolic ratio between energy production and energy consumption in the muscle often results in myoglobinuria (Okafor 2005). The most common symptoms of rhabdomyolysis are muscle pain, weakness, sensitivity, stiffness, and occasionally contractures. In a study, Gabow et al. (1982) found that 50% of patients with rhabdomyolysis showed symptoms that primarily affected the muscles of the thighs, calves, and back. The muscles were swollen and sensitive to palpation.

Other optional symptoms include general malaise, fever, tachycardia, nausea, and vomiting. The associated electrolyte disturbances can lead to restlessness, confusion, and reduced urine output. Dark, typically brown urine is often the first indication of existing rhabdomyolysis. The cause of this color change is existing myoglobinuria. However, it has also been reported that 26% of patients with rhabdomyolysis did not have myoglobinuria (McCarron et al. 1979).

In victims of a lightning strike who show rhabdomyolysis as a result of the accident, early therapy can prevent the development of acute kidney failure. The treatment of these patients consists of fluid intake, alkalinization of the urine, diuretic therapy, correction of electrolyte disturbances, dialysis, and supportive therapy (Okafor 2005; Dall'Aglio et al. 2020). Large amounts of fluid should be administered to maintain adequate urine output. The rate of fluid administration depends on the severity of the myoglobinuria (Honda 1983; Okafor 2005). The goal of fluid intake is a diuresis of at least 3 ml/kg/h and myoglobin-free urine (Dall'Aglio et al. 2020; Okafor 2005). In patients who have survived the complications of a lightning strike and overcome myoglobinuria, the prognosis for a complete recovery of previous kidney function is good in most cases (Okafor 2005).

Case Study

A 36-year-old man was severely injured by a direct lightning strike in Northern Ireland while escorting two children home from school. He suffered an immediate respiratory and cardiac arrest. Witnesses to the accident immediately began resuscitation measures, which were continued by an alerted rescue team upon their arrival at the scene. The first documented heart rhythm was a pulseless electrical activity that turned into ventricular fibrillation. After transport to the emergency department of a clinic, spontaneous return of circulation occurred 50 minutes after the accident. The combination of lightning strike and prolonged resuscitation phase had caused severe metabolic acidosis, hypoxic brain damage, and multipleorgan failure. Skin burns were found on the left side of the neck and on the right big toe. Upon his arrival in the intensive care unit, repeated resuscitation measures were necessary. Due to significant rhabdomyolysis with greatly increased creatine kinase (10,264 U/L with a reference range of 40–320 U/L) and hyperkalemia, renal replacement therapy was initiated. The patient developed acute respiratory distress syndrome and was mechanically ventilated. On the 3rd day, he remained in multiple organ failure with persistently elevated serum lactate levels. He was too unstable for a CT scan transfer. Subsequently, limited fasciotomies of the right upper and lower extremities were performed. An exploratory laparotomy revealed a liver injury, which was managed by compressive wrapping of the liver with abdominal towels ("packing"). On the 4th day, the liver packs were removed and the liver injuries were closed. The patient was then weaned off the inotropes. On the 6th day, a CT scan of his brain and spine was possible. It showed a left temporal ischemia, a small subarachnoid hemorrhage, and a loss of differentiation between gray and white matter as an indication of hypoxic brain damage. An MRI scan of the brain confirmed these findings. The spinal cord was uninjured. After the victim's condition stabilized, a tracheostomy was performed on the 11th day. After recovery of kidney function, dialysis was discontinued after 20 days. As the patient showed pronounced general weakness, neurological examinations followed, which showed a peripheral neuropathy with axonal loss of motor and sensory fibers. A muscle biopsy performed showed a patchy neurogenic myopathy with numerous preserved muscle fibers under electron microscopy. After a period of confusion, the patient made slow progress with intensive multidisciplinary rehabilitation. The tracheostomy was removed after 33 days and after 49 days the man was transferred from the intensive care unit to a regular ward. Twelve weeks after the lightning strike accident, he was transferred to the regional department for patients with brain injuries and was discharged home 26 weeks after the accident. Although healing was progressing, the patient still suffered from persistent weakness and used a walking stick. His skin wounds had healed without surgical intervention (Sleihwah et al. 2018). ◀

Characteristics of the Most Common Renal Complication After Lightning Strike

- After a lightning strike accident, the victim may develop rhabdomyolysis.
- Rhabdomyolysis and myoglobinuria pose the risk of acute renal failure.
- The treatment of this complication of a lightning strike consists of fluid intake, alkalinization of the urine, diuretic treatment, correction of electrolyte disorders, dialysis, and possibly supportive treatment.
- After surviving the complications of the accident, the kidneys have a good chance of recovery.

6.2.9 Pregnancy

Lightning accidents involving pregnant women are extremely rare events. At least 15 case reports can be found in the medical literature (Chan and Sivasamboo 1972, Galster et al. 2016; Graber et al. 1996; Guha-Ray 1979; Pierce et al. 1986; Rees 1965; Weinstein 1979). In all accidents, the mother survived. In 6 cases, an intrauterine fetal death was the result of the accident, in one case the child died a few hours after birth, the other 8 children survived the event. Fetal death is said to have occurred particularly due to the subsequent ended asystole of the mother. However, in the media there is also a lightning accident in which both the death of a pregnant mother and the unborn child are reported (Yoder 2012).

Case Example

In an accident in August in the early 1990s in Baden-Württemberg (Germany), lightning struck a group of trees on the grounds of a well-attended public swimming pool. Four adults and four children, who were under trees at the time, were injured. A 28-year-old man died at the scene of the accident. Among the other 7 victims was a 41-year-old woman who was 6 months pregnant. When an anesthetist and an anesthesia nurse, who also happened to be among the approximately 1200 visitors to the swimming pool, arrived at the woman, she was comatose and had dilated, unresponsive pupils, cardiac arrest, and burns on her neck. The two helpers immediately began chest compressions and mouth-to-mouth resuscitation. Intubation took place about 10 minutes after the lightning strike. The ECG initially showed an asystole, but shortly thereafter a sinus rhythm. After that, the pulse was palpable again, even without the administration of drugs. After the accident victim began to move, she was sedated due to the impending helicopter transport. In the clinic, the death of the fetus was determined. Apart from a unilateral tympanic membrane rupture, which was treated with a tympanoplasty, no further injuries were found.

Two years after the event, the woman still complained of persistent hearing loss on the affected side and showed post-traumatic stress disorder due to the miscarriage she had suffered. Retrograde amnesia for the time of the accident and the days before and after persisted (Graber et al. 1996). ◀

▶ **Note** In the event of a lightning strike accident involving a pregnant woman, the life of the fetus is much more at risk than the life of the expectant mother.

6.2.10 Digestive Tract

After a lightning strike accident, injuries in the area of the digestive tract are very rare. In isolated cases, liver ruptures, gastric perforations, mucosal tears of the esophagus, or stress ulcers of the stomach have been described (Graber et al. 1996; Kilbas et al. 2008; Ohashi et al. 2001; Sleihwah et al. 2018; Wankhede and Sariya 2013). It must also be considered that some of the mentioned injuries could also be caused by intensive resuscitation measures and are therefore not necessarily attributable to a lightning strike (Buschmann and Tsokos 2008).

Injuries in the digestive tract usually require surgical therapies and have good chances of healing with timely diagnosis and treatment.

▶ **Note** After a lightning strike, injuries to the digestive tract are rare. Liver ruptures or gastric perforations require rapid surgical therapy.

6.2.11 Endocrine System

In the literature, there are also cases of lightning accidents with consequences for the human endocrine system. For example, Qureshi (1995) reports on a 27-year-old woman who suffered ear injuries with hearing loss and tinnitus while on the phone during a thunderstorm. An additional functional disorder was a change in her menstrual cycle. While the patient had a 30-day cycle before the accident, this shortened to 23 days after the event. After 3 months, the original cycle spontaneously returned.

Other accident victims reported menstrual disorders that lasted 1-2 years. Furthermore, amenorrhea, premature onset of menopause, decreased libido, or impotence have also occurred after lightning strikes. Damage to the pituitary or hypothalamus is discussed as a cause (O'Keefe Gatewood and Zane 2004).

6.2.12 Other Localizations

The literature also includes individual cases with unusual consequences of a lightning strike accident for a person's health. Representing this group is the occurrence of a central salt loss syndrome. After a direct hit to the head of a 16-year-old boy in Turkey, which immediately rendered the teenager unconscious, the victim developed dehydration and hyponatremia as signs of a central salt loss syndrome. The boy showed fresh bleeding in the cerebral cortex of the right parietal lobe on MRI. After substitution of sodium and fluid, there was a rapid regression, so that the patient could be discharged home on the 5th day after the accident with unremarkable laboratory values (Emet et al. 2010).

▶ **Note** The treatment of victims of a severe lightning accident is carried out by an interdisciplinary team. The most common specialties involved are anesthesia and intensive care, cardiology, neurology, psychiatry, ENT, ophthalmology, surgery, and dermatology.

References

Abhinav K, Al-Chalabi A, Hortobagyi T, Leigh PN (2007) Electrical injury and amyotrophic lateral sclerosis: a systematic review of the literature. J Neurol Neurosurg Psychiatry 78:450–453

Abt JL (1985) The pupillary responses after being struck by lightning. JAMA 254:3312

Adler C, Caviness J (1997) Dystonia secondary to electrical injury: surface electromyographic evaluation and implications for the organicity of the condition. J Neurol Sci 148:187–192

Alyan O, Ozdemir O, Tufekcioglu O, Geyik B, Aras D, Demirkan D (2006) Myocardial injury due to lightning strike—a case report. Angiology 57:219–223

Amy BW, McManus WF, Goodwin CW, Pruitt BA (1985) Lightning injury with survival in five patients. JAMA 253:243–245

Andrews CJ (1992) Telephone related lightning injury. Med J Australia 157:823–826

Andrews CJ (1995) Structural changes after lightning strike, with special emphasis on special sense orifices as portals of entry. Semin Neurol 15:296–303

Andrews CJ, Reisner AD (2017) Neurological and neurophysiological consequences of electrical and lightning shock: review and theories of causation. Neural Regen Res 12:677–686

Andrews CJ, Eadie M, ten Duis HJ, Raphael B, Cash R, Fraunfelder F, Meyer M, Bergstrom LV (1992) Pathophysiology of lightning injury. In: Andrews CJ, Cooper MA, Darvenzia M, Mackerras D (Eds) Lightning injuries: electrical, medical, and legal aspects. CRC Press, Boca Raton, pp 71–114

Angerer F, Hoppe U, Schick B (2009) Blitzeinschlag in einen PKW mit Schädigung des Hörorgans. HNO 57:1081–1084

Apfelberg DB, Masters FW, Robinson DW (1974) Pathophysiology and treatment of lightning injuries. J Trauma 14:453–460

Arévalo JM, Lorente JA, Balseiro-Gómez J (1999) Spinal cord injury after electrical trauma treated in a burn unit. Burns 25:449–452

Auer J (2000) Cardiac involvement in lightning strike injury. Clin Cardiol 23:386

Aydin F, Yildrim OT, Dagtekin E, Aydin AH, Aksit E (2018) Acute inferior myocardial infarction caused by lightning strike. Prehosp Disaster Med 33:658–659

Backhaus R, Kirzinger L, Platen S, Kreuzer PM, Kleiter I, Lürding R, Zack F, Schulte-Mattler W, Schalke B (2016) Blitzschlagverletzungen. Klin Neurophysiol 47:78–84

Baqain E, Haertsch P, Kennedy P (2004) Complete recovery following a high voltage electrical injury associated with delayed onset of quadriplegia and multiple cranial nerves dysfunction. Burns 30:603–605

Bariar LM, Ahmad I, Aggarwal A, Menon RK (2002) Myelopathy following high voltage electrical injury: a case report. Burns 28:699–700

Baxter CR (1970) Present concepts in the management of major electrical injury. Surg Clin North Am 50:1401–1418

Belsole RJ, Smith AA (1990) Reflex sympathetic dystrophy: gate closed by lightning. J Hand Surg 15:523

Bergstrom L, Neblett LW, Sando I, Hemenway WG, Harrison GD (1974) The lightning-damaged ear. Arch Otolaryngol 100:117–121

Bhargava AN, Kasundra GM, Khichar S, Bhushan BS (2014) Lightning strike-induced brachial plexopathy. J Neurosci Rural Pract 5:399–400

Blanchard EB, Hickling EJ, Taylor AE, Loos WR, Forneris CA, Jaccard J (1996) Who develops PTSD from motor vehicle accidents? Behav Res Ther 34:1–10

Blumenthal R (2005) Lightning fatalities on the South African Highveld: a retrospective descriptive study for the period 1997 to 2000. Am J Forensic Med Pathol 26:66–69

Blumenthal R (2021) Injuries and deaths from lightning. J Clin Pathol 74:279–284

Blumenthal R, Saayman G (2017) Case report: lightning-induced pneumomediastinum. Am J Forensic Med Pathol 38:94–96

Blumenthal R, Jandrell IR, West NJ (2012) Does a sixth mechanism exist to explain lightning injuries? Am J Forensic Med Pathol 33:222–226

Bowsher D (1995) The management of central post-stroke pain. Postgrad Med J 71:598–604

Bozan N, Kiroglu AF, Ari M, Turan M, Cankaya H (2016) Tympanic membrane perforation caused by thunderbolt strike. J Craniofac Surg 27:e723–e724

Bremer L (2024) Retrospektive Analyse einer historischen Fallsammlung von letalen Unfällen durch Blitzschlag in der Bundesrepublik Deutschland im Zeitraum 1951–1965 aus rechtsmedizinischer Sicht. Med Diss. Universität Rostock, Rostock

Breugem CC, Van Hertum W, Groenevelt F (1999) High voltage electrical injury leading to a delayed onset tetraplegia, with recovery. Ann N Y Acad Sci 888:131–136

Browne BJ, Gaasch WR (1992) Electrical injuries and lightning. Emerg Med Clin North Am 10:211–229
Brumback R, Feeback DL, Leech RW (1995) Rhabdomyolysis following electrical injury. Semin Neurol 15:329–334
Bryan BC, Andrews CJ, Hurley RA, Taber KH (2009) Electrical injury, part I: mechanisms. J Neuropsychiat Clin Neurosci 21:241–244
Burda CD (1966) Electrocardiographic changes in lightning stroke. Am Heart J 72:521–524
Buschmann C, Tsokos M (2008) Iatrogene Traumata nach frustraner Reanimation. Dtsch Med Wochenschr 133:1244–1248
Butler ED, Grant TD (1977) Electrical injuries, with special reference to the upper extremities. Am J Surg 134:95–101
Cahill KC, Tiong WH, Conroy FJ (2014) Trineural injury to the right hand after domestic electrocution. J Burn Care Res 35:e353–e356
Caksen H, Yuca SA, Demirtas I, Odabas D, Cesur Y, Demirok A (2004) Right thalamic hemorrhage resulting from high-voltage electrical injury: a case report. Brain Dev 26:134–136
Carrera-Izquierdo E, Moran-Sanchez JC, Carrera-Izquierdo M, Jimenez-Corral C, Rodriguez-Recio FJ, Ocastegui-Candial JL (2004) Intracranial haemorrhage secondary to a lightning strike: a case report. Rev Neurol 39:530–532
Chan YF, Sivasamboo R (1972) Lightning accidents in pregnancy. J Obstet Gynaecol Br Commonw 79:761–762
Cherington M (1995) Central nervous system complications of lightning and electrical injuries. Semin Neurol 15:233–240
Cherington M (2003) Neurologic manifestations of lightning strikes. Neurology 60:182–185
Cherington M, Yarnell P, Hallmark D (1993) MRI in lightning encephalopathy. Neurology 43:1437–1438
Cherington M, Yarnell PR, Todd HM (1994) Lightning injury and glioma. Int J Care Inj 25:687–688
Cherington M, Yarnell PR, London SF (1995) Neurologic complications of lightning injuries. West J Med 162:413–417
Cherington M, Krider EP, Yarnell PR, Breed DW (1997) A bolt from the blue: lightning strike to the head. Neurology 48:683–686
Cherington M, Wachtel H, Yarnell PR (1998) Could lightning injury be magnetically induced? Lancet 351:1788
Cherington M, Kurtzman R, Krider EP, Yarnell PR (2001) Mountain medical mystery. Unwitnessed death of a healthy young man, caused by lightning. Am J Forensic Med Pathol 22:296–298
Chia BL (1981) Electrocardiographic abnormalities and congestive cardiac failure due to lightning stroke. Cardiology 68:49–53
Chico MS, Capelli-Schellpfeffer M, Kelley KM, Lee RC (1999) Management and coordination of postacute medical care for electrical trauma survivors. Ann N Y Acad Sci 888:334–342
Christensen JA, Sherman RT, Balis GA, Waumett JD (1980) Delayed neurological injury secondary to high voltage current, with recovery. J Trauma 20:166–168
Clouston P (1995) Central conduction abnormalities after electrical injury. Muscle Nerve 18:675
Cooper MA (1980) Lightning injuries: prognostic signs of death. Ann Emerg Med 9:134–138
Cooper MA (1995) Emergent care of lightning and electrical injuries. Semin Neurol 15:268–278
Cooper MA, Holle RL (2019) Reducing lightning injuries worldwide. Springer, Cham
Cooper MA, Andrews CJ, Holle RL, Lopez R (2001) Lightning injuries. In: Auerbach PS (ed) Wilderness medicine: management of wilderness and environmental emergencies. 4th edn. Mosby, St. Louis, pp 74–76

Cooper MA, Andrews CJ, Holle RL, Blumenthal R, Navarette-Aldana N (2017) Lightning-related injuries and safety. In: Auerbach P, Cushing T, Harris N (eds) Auerbach's wilderness medicine. 7th edn. Elsevier, Philadelphia, pp 71–117

Cooray V, Cooray C, Andrews CJ (2007) Lightning caused injuries in humans. J Electrostatics 65:386–394

Courtman SP, Wilson PM, Mok Q (2003) Case report of a 13-year-old struck by lightning. Paediatr Anaesth 13:76–79

Cwinn AA, Cantrill SV (1985) Lightning injuries. J Emerg Med 2:379–388

Dall'Aglio A, Kissling S, Vollenweider P, Jaccard E (2020) Rhabdomyolysis: early management. Rev Med Suisse 16:2272–2278

Danielson JR, Capelli-Schellpfeffer M, Lee RC (2000) Upper extremity electrical injury. Hand Clin 16:225–234

Davidson GS, Deck JH (1988) Delayed myelopathy following lightning strike: a demyelinating process. Acta Neuropathol 77:104–108

Davis C, Engeln A, Johnson EL, McIntosh SE, Zafren K, Islas AA, McStay C, Smith WR, Cushing T (2014) Wilderness medical society practice guidelines for the prevention and treatment of lightning injuries: 2014 update. Wilderness Environ Med 25:86–95

Demun E, Redd J, Buchanan K, Brennan T, Rowlingson J, Himel H, Morgan R, Edlich R (1993) Reflex sympathetic dystrophy after minor electric shock. J Emerg Med 11:393–396

Desai B, Fairclough R (2011) A case of a speech impediment following a near lightning strike. Int J Em Med 4:60

Deutsche Gesellschaft für Allgemeinmedizin und Familienmedizin (2014) Ohrenschmerzen. S2k-Leitlinie, AWMF-Registernr. 053/009. https://register.awmf.org/assets/guidelines/053-009l_S2k_Ohrenschmerzen_2014-12-abgelaufen.pdf. Accessed: 24 Jan 2023.

Deutsche Gesellschaft für Verbrennungsmedizin (2021) Behandlung thermischer Verletzungen des Erwachsenen. S2k-Leitlinie, AWMF-Registernr. 044-001. https://register.awmf.org/assets/guidelines/044-001l_S2k_Behandlung-thermischer-Verletzungen-des-Erwachsenen_2021-07.pdf. Accessed: 12 Jan 2023.

Deveci M, Bozkurt M, Sengezer M (2001) Clonus: an unusual delayed neurological complication in electrical burn injury. Burns 27:647–651

Dhillon PS, Gupta M (2015) Ophthalmic manifestation postlightning strike. BMJ Case Rep. https://doi.org/10.1136/bcr-2014-207594. Accessed: 29 Jan 2023.

Dinakaran S, Desai SP, Elsom DM (1998) Telephon-mediated lightning injury causing cataract. Injury 29:645–646

Dopkin BH (2003) The clinical science of neurological rehabilitation, 2nd edn. Oxford University Press, Oxford

Dronacahrya L, Poudel R (2008) Lightning induced atrial fibrillation. Kathmandu Univ Med J 6:514–515

Duff K, McCaffrey RJ (2001) Electrical injury and lightning injury: a review of their mechanisms and neuropsychological, psychiatric, and neurological sequelae. Neuropsychol Rev 11:101–106

Duke-Elder S, McFaul PA (1972) Part 2 Non-mechanical injuries. In: Duke-Elder S (ed) System of opthalmology: injuries. vol 14. Mosby, St. Louis, pp 828–834

Dundon BK, Puri R, Leong DP, Worthley MI (2008) Takotsubo cardiomyopathy following lightning strike. Emerg Med J 25:460–461

Duppel H, Löbermann M, Reisinger EC (2009) Aus heiterem Himmel vom Blitz getroffen. Dtsch Med Wochenschr 134:1214–1217

Dutta B (2016) Lichtenberg figure and lightning. Indian J Dermatol 61:109–111

Dwyer JR, Uman MA, Rassoul HK, Al-Dayeh M, Caraway L, Jerauld J, Rakov VA, Jordan DM, Rambo KJ, Corbin V, Wright B (2003) Energetic radiation produced during rocket-triggered lightning. Science 299:694–697

Eber B, Himmel G, Schubert B, Zeuschner J, Dusleag J, Seerainer C, Antoni H, Gasser R, Lind P, Eber O, Klein W (1989) Myokardiale Schädigung nach Blitzschlag. Z Kardiol 78:402–404

Ekoe JM, Cunnigham M, Jaques O, Balgue F, Baumann RP, Humair L, de Torrente A (1985) Disseminated intravascular coagulation and acute myocardial necrosis caused by lightning. Intensive Care Med 11:160–162

Elsom DM (2000) Deaths and injuries caused by lightning in the United Kingdom: analysis of two databases. Atmos Res 56:325–334

Emet M, Caner I, Cakir M, Aslan S, Cakir Z (2010) Lightning injury may cause abrupt cerebral salt wasting syndrome. Am J Emerg Med 28:640.e1-640.e3

Engrav LH, Gottlieb JR, Walkinshaw MD, Heimbach DM, Trumble TE, Grube BJ (1990) Outcome and treatment of electrical injury with immediate median and ulnar nerve palsy at the wrist: a retrospective review and a survey of members of the American Burn Association. Ann Plast Surg 25:166–168

Epperly TD, Stewart JR (1989) The physical effects of lightning injury. J Fam Pract 29:267–272

Erkin G, Akinbingöl M, Uysal H, Keles I, Aybay C, Ozel S (2007) Delayed cervical spinal cord injury after high voltage electrical injury: a case report. J Burn Care Res 28:905–908

Espaillat A, Janigian R, To K (1999) Cataracts, bilateral macular holes, and rhegmatogenous retinal detachment induced by lightning. Am J Ophthalmol 127:216–217

Fan KW, Zhu ZX, Den ZY (2005) An experimental model of an electrical injury to the peripheral nerve. Burns 31:731–736

Farrell D, Starr A (1968) Delayed neurological sequelae of electrical injuries. Neurology 18:601–606

Fidan V, Fidan T, Saracoglu KT (2012) Lightning strike: a rare cause of incudostapedial disruption with intact membrane. Pediatr Emerg Care 28:213–214

Forster SA, Silva IM, Ramos MI, Gragnani A, Ferreira LM (2013) Lightning burn—review and case report. Burns 39:e8–e12

Freeman CB, Goyal M, Bourque PR (2004) MR imaging findings in delayed reversible myelopathy from lightning strike. Am J Neuroradiol 25:851–853

Frommberger U, Angenendt J, Dreßing H (2013) Begutachtung. In: Maercker A (ed) Posttraumatische Belastungsstörungen. 4th edn. Springer, Heidelberg, pp 121–145

Frommberger U, Angenendt J, Berger M (2014) Posttraumatische Belastungsstörung—eine diagnostische und therapeutische Herausforderung. Dtsch Arztebl Int 111:59–65

Fu PK, Hsu HY, Wang PY (2008) Delayed reversible motor neuronopathy caused by electrical injury. J Chin Med Assoc 71:152–154

Gabow PA, Kaehny WD, Kelleher SP (1982) The spectrum of rhabdomyolysis. Medicine 61:141–152

Gallagher JP, Talbert OR (1991) Motor neuron syndrome after electric shock. Acta Neurol Scand 83:79–82

Galster K, Hodnick R, Berkeley RP (2016) Lightning strike in pregnancy with fetal injury. Wilderness Environ Med 27:287–290

Gathier JC (1988) Neurological changes in a soldier struck by lightning. Psych Neurol Neurochirurg 63:195–200

Geary SP, Spencer T, Tilney PVR (2015) A 26-year-old man struck by lightning. Air Med J 34:8–11

Ghosh D, Gupta A, Kohli A (1995) Electrical injury: cervical myelopathy with late onset progressive motor neuron disease. Aust NZ J Med 25:263–264

Gilbert G (1994) Lightning-induced robotic speech. Neurology 44:991–992
Girard P, Jacquot A (1954) Polyneuro-radiculite de type Guillain-Barre a forme acrodynique survenue dans les suites d'une fulguration. Lyon Med 191:209–214
Gluncic I, Roje Z, Gluncic V, Poljak K (2001) Ear injuries caused by lightning: report of 18 cases. J Laryngol Otol 115:4–8
Gordon MA, Silverstein H, Willcox TO, Rosenberg SI (1995) Lightning injury of the tympanic membrane. Am J Otol 16:373–376
Gouse M, Arockiaraj J, Khanapur R, Srinivasan G (2015) Transient paraplegia in an elderly due to lightning injury: an unusual cause. J Emerg Trauma Shock 8:238–239
Graber J, Ummenhofer W, Herion H (1996) Lightning accident with eight victims: a case report and brief review of the literature. J Trauma 40:288–290
Greenberger D, Padesky CA (2015) Mind over Mood, 2nd edn. Guilford Publications, New York
Grubb BP, Karabin B (2007) New onset postural tachycardia syndrome following lightning injury. Pacing Clin Electrophysiol 30:1036–1038
Guardiola B, Planella M, Ferreruela M, Velasco J, Perez-Barcena J, Llompart-Pou J (2010) Lesion cerebral por fulguracion. Med Intens 37:367–368
Guha-Ray DK (1979) Fetal death at term due to lightning. Am J Obstet Gynecol 134:103–105
Halldorsson A, Couch MH (2004) Pneumomediastinum caused by a lightning strike. J Trauma 57:196–197
Hanson GC, McIlwraith GR (1973) Lightning injury: two case histories and a review of management. Br Med J 4:271–274
Harris K, Morris RE, Patel HR, Oltmanns MH (2019) Bilateral ocular injury from lightning strike. Retina 39:e51–e52
Harwood SJ, Catrou PG, Cole GW (1978) Creatin phosphokinase isoenzyme fractions in the serum of a patient struck by lightning. Arch Intern Med 138:645–646
Hawkes CH, Thorpe JW (1992) Acute polyneuropathy due to lightning injury. J Neurol Neurosurg Psychiatry 55:388–390
Hayashi M, Yamada H, Aqatsuma T, Nomura H, Kitahara O (2005) A case of takotsubo-shaped hypokinesis of the left ventricle caused by a lightning strike. Int Heart J 46:933–938
Hegner CF (1917) Lightning—some of its effects. Ann Surg 65:401–409
Heilbronner RL, Pliskin NH (1999) Psychological issues in the neurorehabilitation of electrical injuries. NeuroRehabilitation 13:127–132
Herold G und Mitarbeiter (2017) Innere Medizin. Herold, Köln
Hey D, Rieder W (1983) Erfolgreiche Laien-Reanimation nach Blitzschlag. Dtsch Med Wochenschr 108:1217–1218
Holle RL, Cooper MA, Navarrete-Aldana N (2021) Lightning injury: Occurence and medical treatment. In: Gomes C (ed) Lightning. Science, engineering, and economic implications for developing countries. Springer, Singapore, pp 263–273
Honda N (1983) Acute renale failure and rhabdomyolysis. Kidney Int 23:888–898
Huan-Jui Y, Chih-Yang L, Huei-Yu L, Po-Chih C (2010) Acute ischemic stroke in low-voltage electrical injury: a case report. Surg Neurol Int 1:83
Igbal SB, Rao SJ, Pyrgos GJ, Haas CJ, Padmanabhan S (2023) Acute inferior ST-elevation myocardial infarction mimicked by direct lightning strike: a case report. Eur Heart J Case Rep 7:1–5
Iranyi J, Orovecz B, Somogyi E, Iranyi K (1962) Das Blitztrauma in neuer Sicht. Münch Med Wochenschr 104:1496–1500
Isao T, Masaki F, Riko N, Seiichi H (2005) Delayed brain atrophy after electrical injury. J Burn Care Rehabil 26:456–458
Jafari H, Couratier P, Camu W (2001) Motor neuron disease after electric injury. J Neurol Neurosurg Psychiatry 71:265–267

Jankovic J, Pardo R (1986) Segmental myoclonus. Clinical and pharmacologic study. Arch Neurol 43:1025–1031
Jellinek S (1903) Elektropathologie: Die Erkrankungen durch Blitzschlag und elektrischen Starkstrom in klinischer und forensischer Darstellung. Enke, Stuttgart
Jitsuiki K, Muramatsu K, Shoda S, Yanagawa Y (2020) Lightning injury caused by a side flash. Am J Med Case Rep 12:538–540
Johansen CK, Welker KM, Lindell EP, Petty GW (2008) Cerebral corticospinal tract injury resulting from high-voltage electrical shock. Am J Neuroradiol 29:1142–1144
Johnstone BR, Harding DL, Hocking B (1986) Telephone-related lightning injury. Med J Aust 144:706–709
Jonas L, Fulda G, Nizze H, Zimmermann R, Gross G, Zack F, Kröning G, Holzhüter G, Haas HJ (2002) Detection of gold particles in the neck skin after lightning stroke with evaporation of an ornamental chain. Ultrastruct Pathol 26:153–159
Jones DT, Ogren FP, Roh LH, Moore GF (1991) Lightning and its effects on the auditory system. Laryngoscope 101:830–834
Jost WH, Schönrock LM, Cherington M (2005) Autonomic nervous system dysfunction in lightning and electrical injuries. NeuroRehabilitation 20:19–23
Junkins EP, Kunkel NC, Kriskovich MD (1999) Lightning strike to the head of a helmeted motorcyclist. Am J Emerg Med 17:213–214
Just T, Kramp B, Pau HW (2002) Blitzschlaginduzierte Verletzungen des Ohres. HNO 50:170–171
Kanitkar S, Roberts AH (1988) Paraplegia in an electrical burn: a case report. Burns Incl Therm Inj 14:49–50
Kannan RY, Chester DL, Titley OG (2004) Combined Bennett's fracture subluxation and scapho-trapezio-trapezoidal dislocation secondary to lightning strike. J Trauma 57:1351–1353
Karadas S, Vuruskan E, Dursun R, Sincer I, Gonullu H, Akkaya E (2013) Myocardial infarction due to lightning strike. J Pak Med Assoc 63:1186–1188
Karobath H, Undt W, Hofschneider H (1971) Zur Wirkung des Blitzschlages auf den Organismus mit besonderer Berücksichtigung der Auswirkungen auf das Herz. Verh Dtsch Ges Inn Med 77:455–457
Katz D, White DK, Alexander MP, Klein RB (2004) Recovery of ambulation after traumatic brain injury. Arch Phys Med Rehab 85:865–869
Kessler RC (2000) Posttraumatic stress disorder: the burden to the individual and to society. J Clin Psychiatry 5:4–12
Kessler RC, Sonnega A, Bromet E, Hughes M, Nelson C (1995) Posttraumatic stress disorder in the National Comorbidity Survey. Arch Gen Psychiatry 52:1048–1060
Khan FY (2009) Rhabdomyolysis: a review of the literature. Neth J Med 67:272–283
Kilbas Z, Akin M, Gorgulu S, Mentes O, Ozturk E, Kozak O, Tufan T (2008) Lightning strike: an unusual etiology of gastric perforation. Am J Emerg Med 26:966.e5-966.e7
Kilic E, Genc H, Aydin Ü, Asik B, Satar B (2017) Variations in otological presentation of lightning strike victims: clinical report of 3 patients. Ulus Travma Acil Cerrahi Derg 23:163–166
Kim CT, Bryant P (2001) Complex regional pain syndrome (type I) after electrical injury: a case report of treatment with continuous epidural block. Arch Phys Med Rehabil 82:993–995
Kirchmair W, Dienstl F (1982) Nach Elektrounfall: Kardiale Überwachung? Dtsch Med Wochenschr 107:857–859
Kleiner JP, Wilkin JH (1978) Cardiac effects of lightning stroke. JAMA 240:2757–2759
Kleinot S, Klachko DM, Keeley KJ (1966) Cardiac effects of lightning injury. S Afr Med J 40:1141–1143

Kleiter I, Luerding R, Diendorfer G, Rek H, Bogdahn U, Schalke B (2007) A lightning strike to the head causing a visual cortex defect with simple and complex visual hallucinations. J Neurol Neurosurg Psychiatry 78:423–426

Kleiter I, Schulte-Mattler W, Schalke B (2008) Blitzunfall—Energieübertragungsmechanismen und medizinische Folgen: Effekte auf das Nervensystem. Dtsch Arztebl 105:224

Knaggs RH (2002) Unusual injuries caused by lightning stroke. Wilderness Environ Med 13:162

Ko SH, Chun W, Kim HC (2004) Delayed spinal cord injury following electrical burns: a 7-year experience. Burns 30:691–695

Kobernick M (1982) Electrical injuries: pathophysiology and emergency management. Ann Emerg Med 11:633–638

Koeppen S (1965) Personenschäden durch Blitzeinwirkung. Med Klin 60:1390–1393

Koller J, Orságh J (1989) Delayed neurological sequelae of high-tension electrical burns. Burns 15:175–178

Kotagel S, Rawlings CA, Chen S, Burris G, Nouri S (1982) Neurologic, psychiatric and cardiovascular complications in children struck by lightning. Pediatrics 70:190–192

Krauland W (1951) Schäden und Todesfälle durch Blitzschlag. Dtsch Zeitschr Gerichtl Med 40:298–312

Kravitz H, Wassermann MJ, Valaitis J, Anzinger RE, Naidu SH (1977) Lightning injury: management of a case with ten-day survival. Am J Dis Child 131:413–415

Kruja J, Kuqo A, Grabova S, Rroji A, Vyshka G (2016) Right hemispheric leukoencephalopathy as an incidental finding following a lightning strike. Maced J Med Sci 4:692–694

Kruse R (1966) Außergewöhnlicher EEG-Befund nach cerebralem Blitztrauma beim Kind. Ein Fall von latenter Epilepsie. Dtsch Z Nervenheilk 188:53–61

Kubilius D, Rimdeika R (2012) Simultaneous lightning injury in a group of people: case report. Burns 38:e9–e12

Lakshminarayanan S, Chokroverty S, Eshkar N, Grewal R (2009) The spinal cord in lightning injury: a report of two cases. J Neurol Sci 276:199–201

Lammertse DP (2005) Neurorehabilitation of spinal cord injuries following lightning and electrical trauma. NeuroRehabilitation 20:9–14

Lea JA (1920) Paresis of accomodation following injury by lightning. Br Ophthalmol 4:417

Lederer W, Wiedermann FJ, Cerchiari E, Baubin MA (2000) Electricity-associated injuries II: outdoor management of lightning-induced casualities. Resuscitation 43:89–93

Leira TLL, Pires LM, Kruse ML, de Lima GG (2013) Struck by lightning: a case of nature-induced pre-excited atrial fibrillation. Circ Arrhythm Electrophysiol 6:e20–e21

Levy DR, Akiyama T (2007) Lightning-induced ventricular fibrillation. Cardiol J 14:91–94

Lichtenberg R, Dries D, Ward K, Marshall W, Scanlon P (1993) Cardiovascular effects of lightning strikes. J Am Coll Cardiol 21:531–536

Lim JK, Lee EH, Chhem RK (2001) Physeal injury in a lightning strike survivor. J Pediatr Orthop 21:608–612

Mahajan A, Rajan R, Regan PJ (2008) Lichtenberg figures: cutaneous manifestation of phone electrocution from lightning. J Plast Reconstr Aesthet Surg 61:111–113

Makin S (2023) Lightning in Brunei: a follow-up of a single strike affecting 29 serving personnel of the Royal Gurkha Rifles. BMJ Mil Health Mar20:e002393.doi:10.1136/military-2023-002393.

Mankani MH, Abramov GS, Boddie A, Lee RC (1994) Detection of peripheral nerve injury in electrical shock patients. Ann N Y Acad Sci 720:206–212

Mann H, Kozic Z, Boulos MI (1983) CT of lightning injury. Am J Neuroradiol 4:976–977

Martelli MF, Zasler ND, Bender MC, Nicholson K (2004) Psychological, neuropsychological, and medical considerations in assessment and management of pain. J Head Trauma Rehabil 19:10–28

Mason AD, Crocett RK (2000) When lightning strikes … a case report and review of the literature. Int Pediatr 15:174–179

Matthews MS, Fahey AL (1997) Plastic surgical considerations in lightning injuries. Ann Plast Surg 39:561–565

McCarron DA, Elliot WC, Rose JS, Bennett WM (1979) Severe mixed metabolic acidosis secondary to rhabdomyolysis. Am J Med 67:905–908

McCrady-Kahn VL, Kahn AM (1981) Lightning burns. West J Med 134:215–219

McIntyre WF, Simpson CS, Redfearn DP, Abdollah H, Baranchuk A (2010) The lightning heart: a case report and brief review of the cardiovascular complications of lightning injury. Indian Pacing Electrophysiol J 10:429–434

Milton WJ, Hal O'Dell R, Warner EG (1996) MRI of lightning injury: early white matter changes associated with cerebral dysfunction. J Okla State Med Assoc 89:93–94

Modayil PC, Lloyd GW, Mallik A, Bowdler DA (2014) Inner ear damage following electric current and lightning injury: a literature review. Eur Arch Otorhinolaryngol 271:855–861

Möhle F, Preuss J, Madea B, Doberentz E (2015) Vier Tage überlebter Blitzschlag nach zunächst erfolgreicher Reanimation. Rechtsmedizin 25:561–565

Moore MC (1956) Ocular injury from lightning current and lightning flash. Trans Ophthalmol Soc Aust 16:87–92

Morgan ZV Jr, Headley RN, Alexander EA, Sawyer CG (1958) Atrial fibrillation and epidural hematoma associated with lightning stroke; report of a case. N Engl J Med 259:956–959

Morris HR, Moriabadi NF, Lees AJ, Dick DJ, Turjanski D (1998) Parkinsonism following electrical injury to the hand. Mov Disord 13:600–602

Moulson AM (1984) Blast injury of the lungs due to lightning. Br Med J 289:1270–1271

Muehlberger T, Vogt PM, Munster AM (2001) The long-term consequences of lightning injuries. Burns 27:829–833

Murty OP (2009) Lightning fatality with blast, flame, heat and current effects: a macroscopic and microscopic view. J Forensic Leg Med 16:162–167

Naik SB, Krishna RVM (2018) A case of keraunoparalysis: a bolt from the blue. Indian J Crit Care Med 22:804–805

Nebuchennykh M, Loseth S, Lindal S, Mellgren SI (2009) The value of skin biopsy with recording of intraepidermal nerve fiber density and quantitative sensory testing in the assessment of small fiber involvement in patients with different causes of polyneuropathy. J Neurol 256:1067–1075

Netchiporouk E, Moreau L, Ramirez LP, Castillo PAC, Bravo FP, Del Solar MC, Sasseville D, Ramos C (2015) Eruptive disseminated pyogenic granulomas following lightning injury. Dermatology 230:199–203

Nield LS, Kamat D (2004) Long-term sequelae of lightning strike in a child: a case report and review. Clin Pediatr 43:563–567

Noel LP, Clarke WN, Addison D (1980) Ocular complications of lightning. J Pediatr Ophthalmol Strabismus 17:245–246

Norman ME, Younge BR (1999) Association of high-dose intravenous methylprednisolone with reversal of blindness from lightning in two patients. Ophthalmology 106:743–745

Norman ME, Albertson D, Younge BR (2001) Ophthalmic manifestations of lightning strike. Surv Ophthalmol 46:19–24

O'Brien CF (1995) Involuntary movement disorders following lightning and electrical injuries. Semin Neurol 15:263–267

Obszanski B, Tulecki L, Kutarski A, Kleinrok A (2019) Lightning-induced pacing system malfunction: a case report. Eur Heart J Case Rep 3:1–5

Offiah C, Heran M, Graeb D (2007) Lightning strike: a rare cause of bilateral ossicular disruption. Am J Neuroradiol 28:974–975

Oflu AT, Kacar E, Pektas A, Bukulmez A (2021) A rare complication of lightning strike: pulmonary contusion. North Clin Istanb 8:619–622

Ohashi M, Hosoda Y, Fujishiro Y, Tuyuki A, Kikuchi K, Obara H, Kitagawa N, Ishikawa T (2001) Lightning injury as a blast injury of skull, brain and visceral lesions: clinical and experimental evidences. Keio J Med 50:257–262

Okafor UV (2005) Lightning injuries and acute renal failure: a review. Ren Fail 27:129–134

O'Keefe Gatewood M, Zane RD (2004) Lightning injuries. Emerg Med Clin North Am 22:369–403

Ondo W (1997) Lingual dystonia following electrical injury. Mov Disord 12:253

Orbak Z, Kara IS (2010) Unusual complication in a child with lightning strike: cerebral salt wasting. Childs Nerv Syst 26:1125–1127

Ozdemir A, Seymen P, Yürekli OA, Caymaz M, Barut Y, Eres M (2002) Transient hypothalamic hypothyroidism and diabetes insipidus after electrical injury. South Med J 95:467–468

Ozgun B, Castillo M (1995) Basal ganglia hemorrhage related to lightning strike. Am J Neuroradiol 16:1370–1371

Palmer ABD (1987) Lightning injury causing prolongation of the Q-T interval. Postgrad Med J 63:891–894

Panagiotis T, Limmroth V, Perbix W, Gerbershagen M, Knam F, Spilker G (2008) Guillain-Barre syndrome after lightning strike. Burns 34:722–726

Paterson JH, Turner JW (1944) Lightning and the central nervous system. J Roy Arm Med Corps 82:73

Patnaik A, Mahapatra AK, Jha M (2015) Pan-brachial plexus neuropraxia following lightning: a rare case report. Surg Neurol Int 6:110–112

Peters WJ (1983) Lightning injury. Can Med Assoc J 128:148–150

Pierce MR, Henderson RA, Mitchell JM (1986) Cardiopulmonary arrest secondary to lightning injury in a pregnant woman. Ann Emerg Med 15:597–599

Pizzi B, Petrucci E, Marinangeli F (2023) Emergency cricothyrotomy in a harsh environment: a case report of complete airway obstruction following a lightning strike. A A Pract 17:e01688

Platen M (1913) Die neue Heilmethode. vol 3. Deutsches Verlagshaus Bong & Co, Berlin

Pliskin N, Capelli-Schellpfeffer M, Law RT, Malina AC, Kelley KM, Lee RC (1998) Neuropsychological symptom presentation after electrical injury. J Trauma 44:709–715

Poser C (1994) Notes on the pathogenesis of multiple sclerosis. Clin Neurosci 2:258–265

Poulsen P, Knudstrup P (1986) Lightning causing inner ear damage and intracranial haematoma. J Laryngol Otol 100:1067–1070

Pradhan E, Khatri A, Ahmed AA, Lama AJ, Khanal R, Bajracharya L, Adhikari S (2020) Lightning injury to eye: brief review of the literature and case series. Clin Ophthalmol 14:597–607

Primeau M (2005) Neurorehabilitation of behavioral disorders following lightning and electrical trauma. NeuroRehabilitation 20:25–33

Primeau M, Engelstatter GH, Bares KK (1995) Behavioral consequences of lightning and electrical injury. Semin Neurol 15:279–285

Pschyrembel W (2020) Klinisches Wörterbuch, 286th edn. De Gruyter, Berlin

Puchstein S (2016) Zur Letalität von Blitzunfällen. Med Diss. Universität Rostock, Rostock

Püschel K, Kalka R, Schulz F, Zack F (2009) Tod durch Blitzschlag-Fahrrad als "(Faraday'sche) Falle". Rechtsmedizin 19:102–104

Quinn N, Maraganore D (2000) Parkinsonism following electrical injury to the hand. Mov Disord 15:587–588
Qureshi NH (1995) Indirect lightning strike via telephone wire. Injury 26:629–630
Rahmani SH, Faridaalaee G, Jahangard S (2015) Acute transient hemiparesis induced by lightning strike. Am J Emerg Med 33:984e1–3
Ramati A, Pliskin NH, Keedy S, Erwin RJ, Fink JW, Bodnar EN, Lee RC, Cooper MA, Kelley K, Sweeney JA (2009) Alteration in functional brain systems after electrical injury. J Neurotrauma 26:1815–1822
Rao KA, Rao LG, Kamath AN, Jain V (2009) Bilateral macular hole secondary to remote lightning strike. Indian J Ophthalmol 57:470–472
Raule P (1986) Tod durch thermische Einwirkungen. In: Forster B (ed) Praxis der Rechtsmedizin. Thieme, Stuttgart New York, pp 197–204
Rees WD (1965) Pregnant woman struck by lightning. Br Med J 1:103–104
Reisner AD (2006) A case of lightning injury with delayed-onset psychiatric and cognitive symptoms. Brain Inj 20:1093–1097
Reisner AD (2013) Possible mechanisms for delayed neurological damage in lightning and electrical injury. Brain Inj 27:565–569
Resnick H, Acierno R, Waldrop AE, King D, Danielson C, Ruggiero KJ, Kilpatrick D (2007) Randomized controlled evaluation of an early intervention to prevent post-rape psychopathology. Behav Res Ther 45:2432–2447
Richards A (1973) Traumatic facial palsy. Proc Roy Soc Med 66:28–29
Ritenour AE, Morton MJ, McManus JG, Barillo DJ, Cancio LC (2008) Lightning injury: a review. Burns 34:585–594
Rosenberg DB (1989) Neurologic sequelae of minor electric burns. Arch Phys Med Rehabil 70:914–915
Saddler MC, Thomas JE (1990) Temporary bulbar palsy following lightning strike. Cent Afr J Med 36:161–162
Scalzitti NJ, Pfannenstiehl TJ (2014) A lightning strike causing a cholesteatoma: a unique form of otologic blast injury. Otol Neurotol 35:e298–e300
Schaidt G (1977) Spuren an Kleidungsstücken beim Blitzunfall. Arch Kriminol 159:93–96
Schniers E (2005) Schädigungen und Tod nach Blitzschlag—eine Synopsis aus rechtsmedizinischer Sicht. Med Diss. Universität Rostock, Rostock
Schwab M, Wiegand H, Bentsen P, Hochrein H (1989) Infarkt-EKG nach Blitzunfall. Z Kardiol 78:611–614
Sellier K (1975) Schäden und Tod durch Elektrizität. In: Mueller B (Hrsg) Gerichtliche Medizin. 2nd edn. Teil 1. Springer, Berlin, pp 538–563
Sener MU, Demir A, Sener A (2019) Lightning-strike-induced acute lung injury: a case report. Ulus Travma Acil Derrahi Derg 25:198–201
Shantha TR (1991) Causalgia induced by telephone-mediated lightning electrical injury and treated by interpleural block. Anesth Analg 73:507–508
Sharma M, Smith A (1978) Paraplegia as a result of lightning injury. Br Med J 2:1464–1465
Silbergleit AK, Trenkner SW (1988) Dysphagia following lightning strike. Dysphagia 2:228–229
Silverside J (1964) The neurological sequelae of electrical injury. Can Med Assoc J 91:195–204
Sinha AK (1985) Lightning-induced myocardial injury. A case report with management. Angiology 36:327–331
Skan DA (1949) Death from lightning-stroke, with multiple injuries. Br Med J 1:666
Sleihwah A, Baker J, Gowers C, Elsom DM, Rashid A (2018) Lightning injuries in Northern Ireland. Ulster Med J 87:168–172

Soltermann B, Frutiger A, Kuhn M (1991) Lightning injury with lung bleeding in a tracheotomized patient. Chest 99:240–242

Spaar FW (1955) Hirnbefund nach Tod durch Blitzschlag. Virchows Arch 326:732–747

Stanley LD, Suss RA (1985) Intracerebral hematoma secondary to lightning stroke: case report and review of the literature. Neurosurgery 16:686–688

Steffen D, Schoneweis D, Nelssen J (1992) Hind limb paralysis from electrical shock in three gilts. J Am Vet Med Assoc 200:812–813

Steinbaum S, Harviel JD, Jaffin JH, Jordan MH (1994) Lightning strike to the head: case report. J Trauma 36:113–115

Stütz N, Weiss D, Reichert B (2006) Verletzungen durch Blitzschlag. Unfallchirurg 109:495–498

St Yves C (1722) Les causes accidentelles, qui peuvent blesser la vue. In: Nouveau traité des maladies des yeux, les remèdes qui y conviennent et les opérations de chiururgie que leurs guérisons exigent. PA Le Mercier, Paris, pp 368–370

Suri ML, Vijayan GP (1978) Neurological sequelae of lightning (a case report). J Assoc Physicians India 26:209–212

Tadler M, Rüegg E, Niquille M, Gencer B, Gautschi OP, Pittet-Cuénod B, Modarressi A (2017) Multi-organ injuries due to a lightning strike: a case report highlighting the importance of a multi-disciplinary approach. Case Reports Plast Surg Hand Surg 4:1–4

Taussig HB (1968) "Death" from lightning—and the possibility of living again. Ann Intern Med 68:1345–1353

ten Duis HJ, Klasen HJ, Reenalda PE (1985) Keraunoparalysis, a 'specific' lightning injury. Burns Incl Therm Inj 12:54–57

Thomas M, Pillai M, Krishna Das KV (1991) Intracranial haematoma resulting from lightning stroke. J Assoc Physicians India 39:421–422

Tibesar RJ, Saswata R, Hom DB (2000) Fracture from a lightning strike injury to the face. Otolaryngol Head Neck Surg 123:647–649

Tribble CG, Persing JA, Morgan RF, Kenney JG, Edlich RF (1985) Lightning injuries. Compr Ther 11:32–40

Turan M, Kalkan F, Bozan N, Özcalimli I, Erdem MZ, Yalinkilic A, Garca MF (2015) Isolated sensorineural hearing loss as a sequela after lightning. Case Rep Otolaryngol. https://doi.org/10.1155/2015/738416. Epub 2015 Jun 16

Umminger JM (2018) Neurologische Langzeitschäden bei Blitzopfern—vergleichende Literaturrecherche zu neurologischen, neuropsychologischen und psychiatrischen Langzeitschäden nach Blitzschlag, deren Behandlung und Prognose. Med Diss. Universität Regensburg, Regensburg

van Ruler R, Eikendal T, Kooij FO, Tan ECTH (2022) A shocking injury: a clinical review of lightning injuries highlighting pitfalls and treatment protocol. Injury 53:3070–3077

van Waes OJF, van de Woestijne PC, Halm JA (2014) "Thunderstruck": penetrating thoracic injury from lightning strike. Ann Emerg Med 63:457–459

Varghese G, Mani MM, Redford JB (1986) Spinal cord injuries following electrical accidents. Paraplegia 24:159–166

Venkateswaran N, Galor A (2018) Rosette-shaped cataract due to lightning injury. JAMA Ophthalmol 136:e175719

Ventura F, Barranco R, Bonsignore A, De Stefano F (2017) A unusual lightning death in an indoor setting. A case report. Am J Forensic Med Pathol 38:1–4

Volinsky JB, Hanson JB, Lustig JV, Tunnessen WW (1994) Clinical picture. Arch Fam Med 3:657–658

Wakasugi C, Masui M (1986) Secondary brain hemorrhages associated with lightning stroke: report of a case. Jap J Legal Med 40:42–46

Wankhede AG, Sariya DR (2013) Damage due to lightning when it strikes the face. Forensic Sci Int 224:e1–e3
Weeramanthri TS, Puddey IB, Beilin LJ (1991) Lightning strike and autonomic failure-coincidence or causally related? J R Soc Med 84:687–688
Weinstein L (1979) Lightning: a rare cause of intrauterine death with maternal survival. South Med J 72:632–633
Werdan K, Boeken U, Briegel MJ, Buerke A, Geppert A, Janssens U, Kelm M, Michels G, Pilarczyk K, Schlitt A, Thiele H, Willems S, Zeymer U, Zwißler B, Delle-Karth G, Ferrari M, Figulla H, Heller A, Hindricks G, Pichler-Cetin E, Pieske BM, Prondzinsky R, Thielmann M, Bauersachs J, Kopp I, Ruß M (2021) Kurzversion der 2. Auflage der deutsch-österreichischen S3-Leitlinie "Infarkt-bedingter kardiogener Schock—Diagnose, Monitoring und Therapie". Anaesthesist 70:42–70
Wetli CV (1996) Keraunopathology. An analysis of 45 fatalities. Am J Forensic Med Pathol 17:89–98
Whitcomb D, Martinez JA, Daberkow D (2002) Lightning injuries. South Med J 95:1331–1334
Wilbourn AJ (1995) Peripheral nerve disorders in electrical and lightning injuries. Semin Neurol 15:241–255
Yarnell PR (2005) Neurorehabilitation of cerebral disorders following lightning and electrical trauma. NeuroRehabilitation 20:15–18
Yoder M (2012) Pregnant amish woman, killed by lightning on due date. July 25, 2012. http://www.huffingtonpost.com/2012/07/25/mary-yoder-pregnant-amish_n_1700500.html. Accessed: 8 Mar 2016
Youngs R, Deck J, Kwok P, Hawke M (1988) Severe sensorineural hearing loss caused by lightning. Arch Otolaryngol Head Neck Surg 114:1184–1187
Zack F, Büttner A (2016) Rechtsmedizinische Aspekte der Lichtenberg-Figuren nach Blitzschlag. Rechtsmedizin 26:425–428
Zack F, Büttner A (2020) Blitzunfall. Teil 2: Pathophysiologische und diagnostische Aspekte bei tödlichen Ereignissen. Rechtsmedizin 30:345–356
Zack F, Hammer U, Klett I, Wegener R (1997) Myocardial injury due to lightning. Int J Legal Med 110:326–328
Zack F, Rothschild MA, Wegener R (2007) Blitzunfall—Energieübertragungsmechanismen und medizinische Folgen. Dtsch Ärztebl 104:A3545–A3549
Zack F, Rammelsberg JO, Graf B, Büttner A (2010) Tod durch Blitzschlag—und wieder unter einem Baum. Rechtsmedizin 20:108–110
Zack F, Raphael T, Kupfer J, Jokuszies A, Vogt PM, Büttner A, Püschel K, Schalke B, Todt M, Dettmeyer R (2013) Vier Todesopfer nach einem Blitzunfall auf einem Golfplatz. Rechtsmedizin 23:114–118
Zack F, Puchstein S, Büttner A (2016) Letalität von Blitzunfällen. Rechtsmedizin 26:9–11
Zasler ND (1996) Neuromedical diagnosis and management of postconcussive disorders. In: Horn LJ, Zasler ND (eds) Medical rehabilitation of traumatic brain injury. Hanley & Belfus, Philadelphia, pp 133–170
Zeana CD (1984) Acute transient myocardial ischemia after lightning injury. Int J Cardiol 5:207–209
Zoccolella S, Masi G, Mezzapesa D, Carnicella F, Iliceto G, Lamberti P, Serlenga L (2008) Motoneuron disease after electric injury: a case report. Neurol Sci 29:47–49

7 Death by Lightning Strike

A person can remain unharmed, be slightly, moderately, or severely injured, or die from a lightning strike, particularly depending on the type of energy transfer (see Chap. 4). The proportion of fatal lightning accidents among all events involving human injuries varies widely according to the literature (see Sect. 7.5). In recent decades, there has been a significant decline in fatal lightning accidents in industrialized countries (Cooper and Holle 2019). While in the USA from 1900–1925 about 3.5–7 people per 1 million inhabitants died from lightning strikes, this rate has continuously decreased to below 1 after 1960 and even below 0.1 in recent years. A similar decline in fatal lightning victims per 1 million inhabitants was also found in Canada and numerous European countries, including Germany (Cooper and Holle 2019; Schniers 2005).

The rarity of fatal lightning accidents, the possibility of events with discrete characteristic findings, lack of knowledge, and insufficient care by the examining physician favor the misrecognition of the correct cause of death (Blanco-Pampin et al. 1997; Ebertz 1891; Pollak 2000; Pollak et al. 1988; Sellier 1975; Zack and Büttner 2020).

Victims of a fatal lightning strike can die at the scene of the accident or after a time interval of up to several weeks. The various pathophysiological processes and the characteristic findings for the correct diagnosis during the external and internal post-mortem examination are presented below. The significant decrease in fatal accidents in recent decades also results in a noteworthy relevance for the professional literature published many years ago on this extraordinary type of accident (Zack and Büttner 2020).

> **Note** Fatal accidents caused by lightning strikes have been repeatedly misidentified by examining physicians.

F. Zack, *Accidents Caused by Lightning Strikes*,
https://doi.org/10.1007/978-3-662-71066-1_7

7.1 External Post-Mortem Examination

Fatal accidents caused by lightning strikes can be divided into observed and unobserved events (Cherington et al. 2001; Cooper et al. 2017). There have repeatedly been problems in making the correct diagnosis in cases of death that were neither witnessed nor observed by injured parties. A misdiagnosis in observed lightning accidents is rare. A fatal lightning accident that occurred in Vienna was particularly noteworthy due to the numerous characteristic findings that the examining physician either misinterpreted or overlooked due to not undressing the victim (Pollak 2000; Pollak et al. 1988).

Case Study

On a humid warm day in May 1987, several forest workers near Vienna (Austria) were erecting a wildlife fence. When heavy rain set in, they finished their work. Suddenly, the workers were blinded by a bright flash of light. At the same moment, a 53-year-old forest worker collapsed lifelessly to the ground. His colleagues immediately began first aid measures, which were unsuccessful. When the emergency doctor arrived at the scene of the accident, he pronounced the forest worker dead. About an hour after the death was confirmed, another doctor conducted a external post-mortem examination as part of police investigations and documented that there were no signs of lightning impact. Based on information from relatives about pre-existing conditions, he suspected a natural death due to cardiac cause.

Despite the stated natural cause of death, a police-ordered autopsy took place about 20 hours after death, during which it was found that the body was still fully clothed after the medical post-mortem examination. The outer work clothes showed no damage. However, the shirt worn underneath was torn several times at the front and in the neck region, with the damages showing rolled and hardened edges. Under the microscope, melting effects were detectable at these locations. A 0.5 mm perforation was found on the upper leather of the left work shoe.

During the external inspection carried out as part of the autopsy, singed body hairs were found in the left parietal-occipital area as well as on the chest and legs. On the outside of the left foot, there was a finger-wide, linear erythema. Several perforations of the skin with gray-white, slightly raised edges were detected on the sole of the left foot. The heart showed no pathomorphological findings (Pollak 2000; Pollak et al. 1988). ◄

In all cases of death where the post-mortem examiner mentions death by lightning strike but is not sure, e.g., in an unobserved event, he should always research the weather for the period of death and consider it in his diagnosis (see Sect. 7.1.5).

7.1.1 Victim's Surroundings

As with any medical post-mortem examination, the examiner's attention should never be solely focused on the deceased person in the case of death by lightning strike. A comprehensive picture of the immediate surroundings of the discovery site can already provide crucial clues to the correct post-mortem diagnosis. The findings that can be useful for the correct diagnosis are diverse. In addition to people injured or killed by lightning strikes, deceased mammals such as horses, dogs, and sheep, or fatally injured birds have been found in the immediate vicinity of the discovered persons (Carte et al. 2002; Jefferiss 1876; Offiah et al. 2007; Schaidt 1977; Spaar 1955) (Fig. 7.1). When people were injured who were under trees at the time of the accident, characteristic bark defects (Fig. 7.2, 7.3 and 7.4), broken branches or split trunks on the trees, as well as burnt grass at the transition from the tree trunk to the ground (Fig. 7.5) could be observed (Zack et al. 1997, 2010, 2013).

Craters up to 2 m in diameter have been observed in the ground after lightning strikes, with stones and sand having been thrown far away (Blumenthal 2022). Buildings under

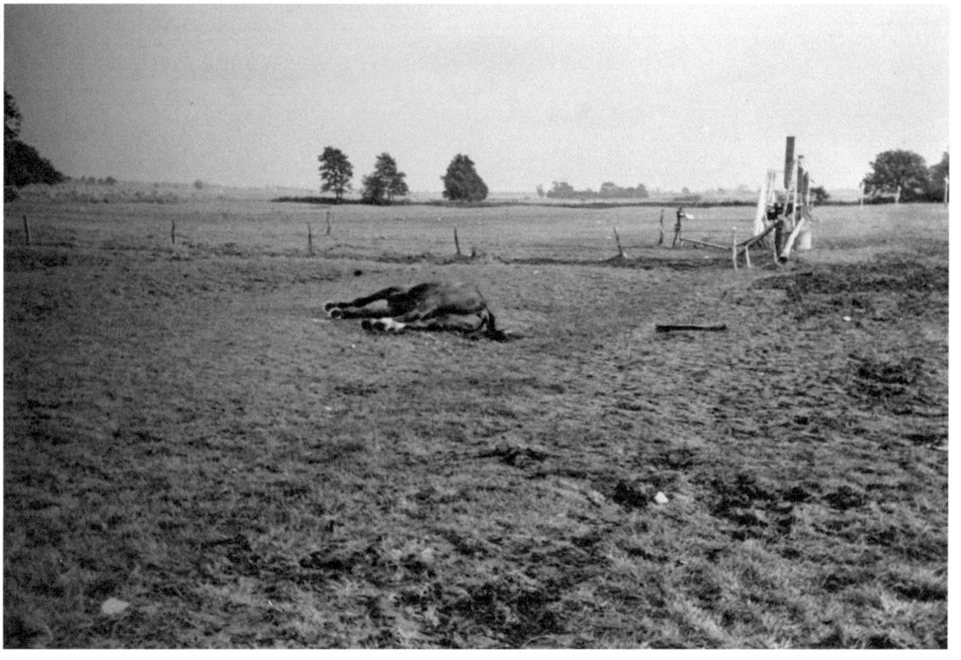

Fig. 7.1 Site of a lightning strike accident, in which both the rider (already brought away) and the horse died. (Historical Collection of the Committee for Lightning Rod Construction for the United Economic Area e. V.)

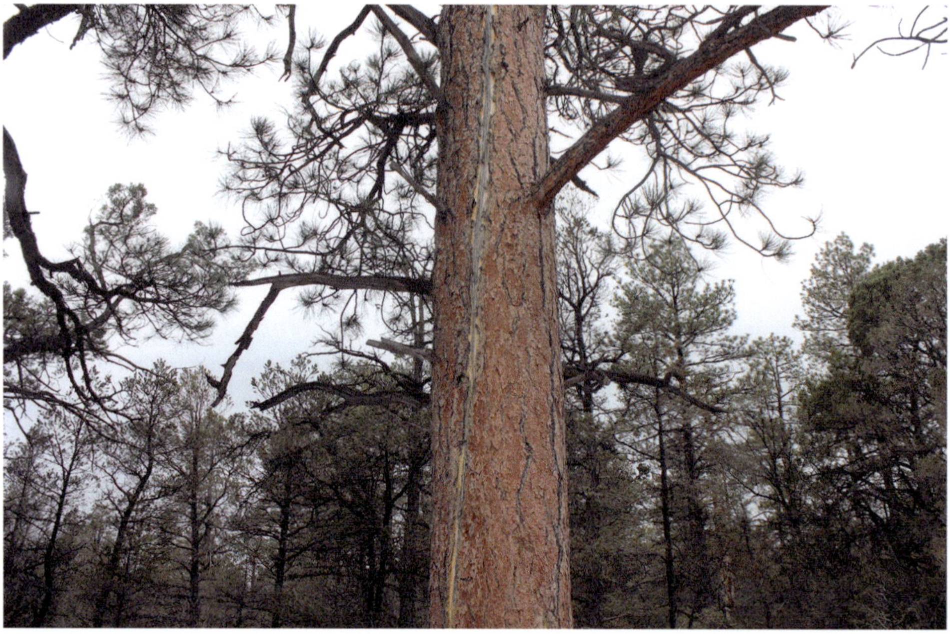

Fig. 7.2 Nearly vertical bark defect of a pine after a lightning strike. (Own illustration)

construction, huts, shelters, and other places where people sought shelter from the rain and were injured by lightning, subsequently showed property damage such as wall destruction, shattered wooden beams, or fire damage (Zack et al. 2013) (Fig. 7.6, 7.7 and 7.8). In other lethal accidents caused by lightning, crater-like torn-out parts of a stony sidewalk next to a pedestrian and numerous detached parts of the bitumen surface of the road next to a cyclist were observed (Blumenthal 2012; Püschel et al. 2009).

> **Note** Lethal accidents caused by lightning often go hand in hand with lightning-related damage to objects or animals killed in the immediate vicinity of the victim.

A medical examiner noted a nearby plastic bag with thermal damage in the form of scorch marks at the scene of a fatal lightning accident in Germany, on the beach of the Baltic Sea. Inside the bag were two aluminum knives, the backs of which had fused together (Schniers 2005). In a fatal lightning accident involving a man who had died in bed in an isolated older house in the countryside in Spain, the medical examiner overlooked numerous thermally induced perforations in the insulation of the surface-mounted wiring in the bedroom, as well as a similarly caused perforation in the headboard of the victim's wooden bed (see Chap. 4) (Blanco-Pampin et al. 1997). Furthermore, Lichtenberg figures on golf turf, sidewalk slabs, or other objects indicate a lightning strike (Cherington et al. 2003; Weimann and Prokop 1963; Zack and Büttner 2020). In a fatal

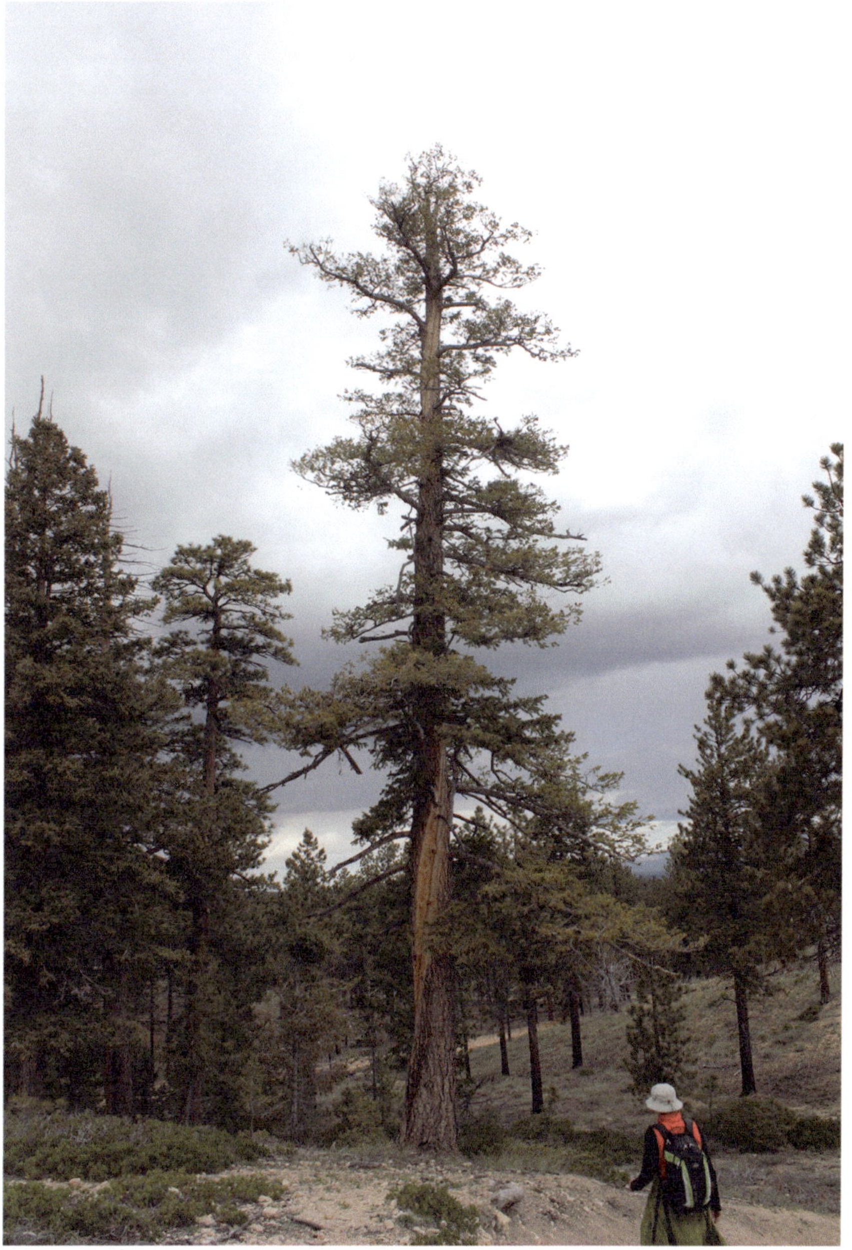

Fig. 7.3 Spiral bark defect of a pine after a longer past lightning strike. (Own illustration)

lightning accident involving an angler, his boat subsequently showed lightning-related thermal damage (Lifschultz and Donoghue 1993a). In a retrospective analysis of 235 fatal lightning events in Germany, findings in the immediate vicinity of the accident site

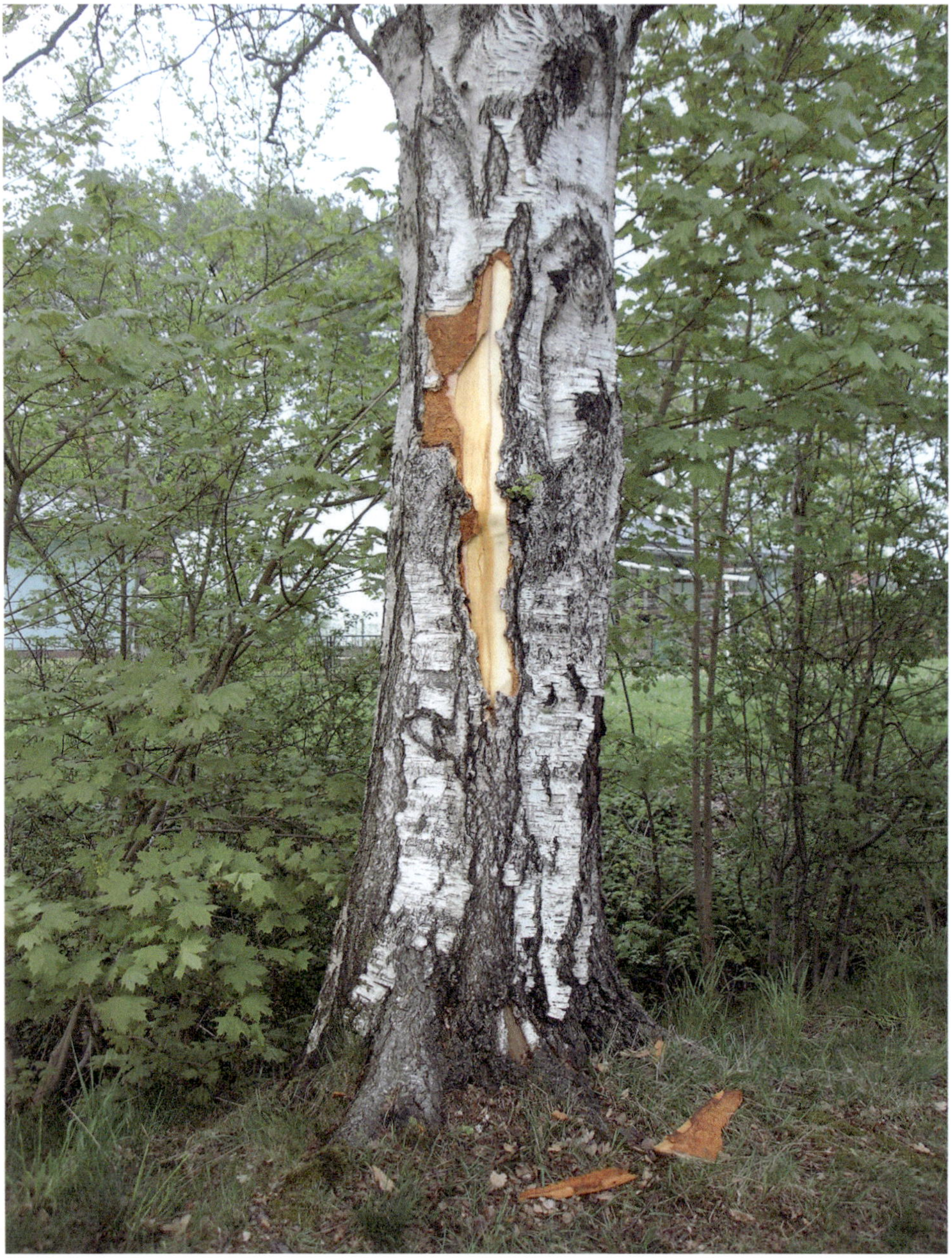

Fig. 7.4 Area-wide fresh bark splintering on a birch after a lightning strike. (Own illustration)

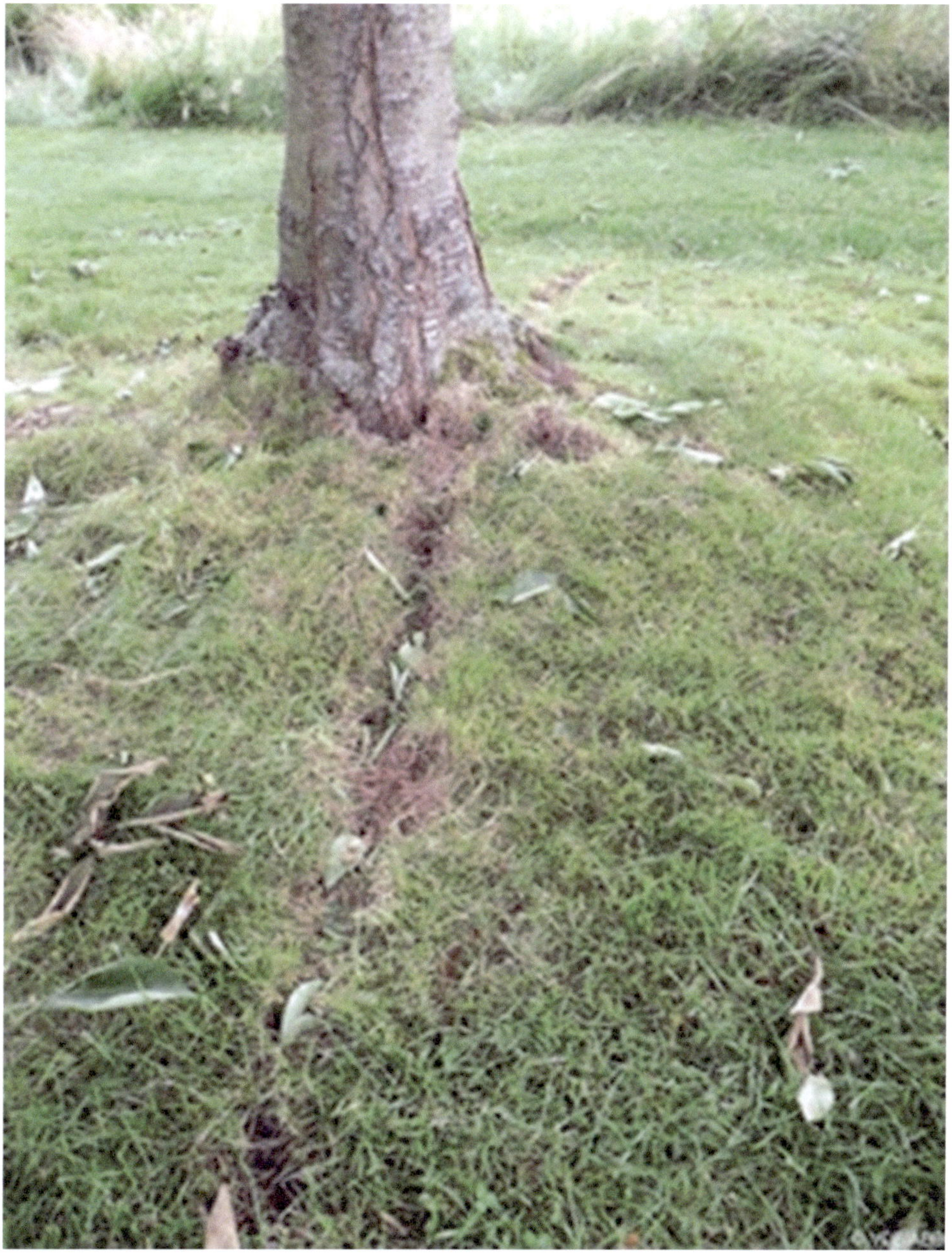

Fig. 7.5 Trace of the lightning channel from a cherry tree over the grass turf to four accident victims on a golf course. (Photo with kind permission: Thomas Raphael)

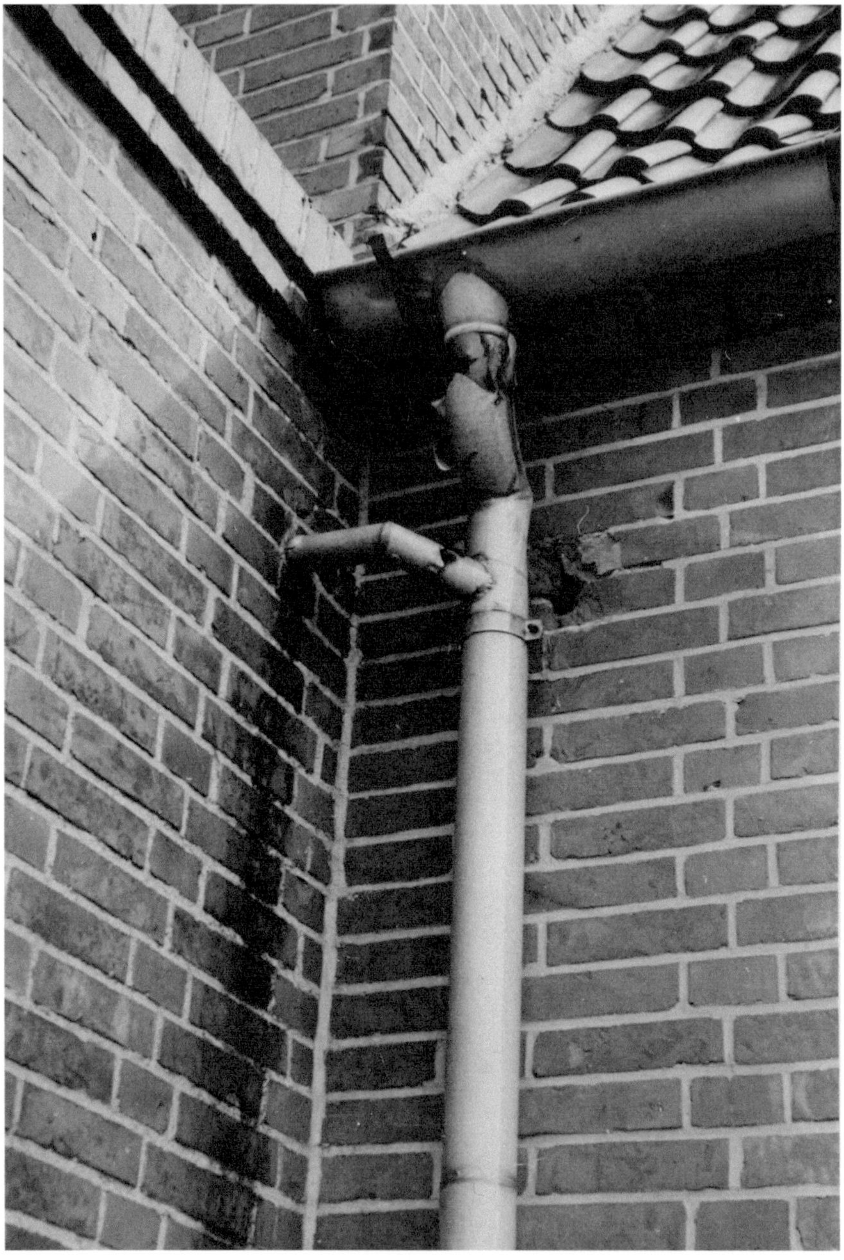

Fig. 7.6 Wall and downpipe of a house damaged by a lightning strike. (Historical Collection of the Committee for Lightning Conductor Construction for the United Economic Area e. V.)

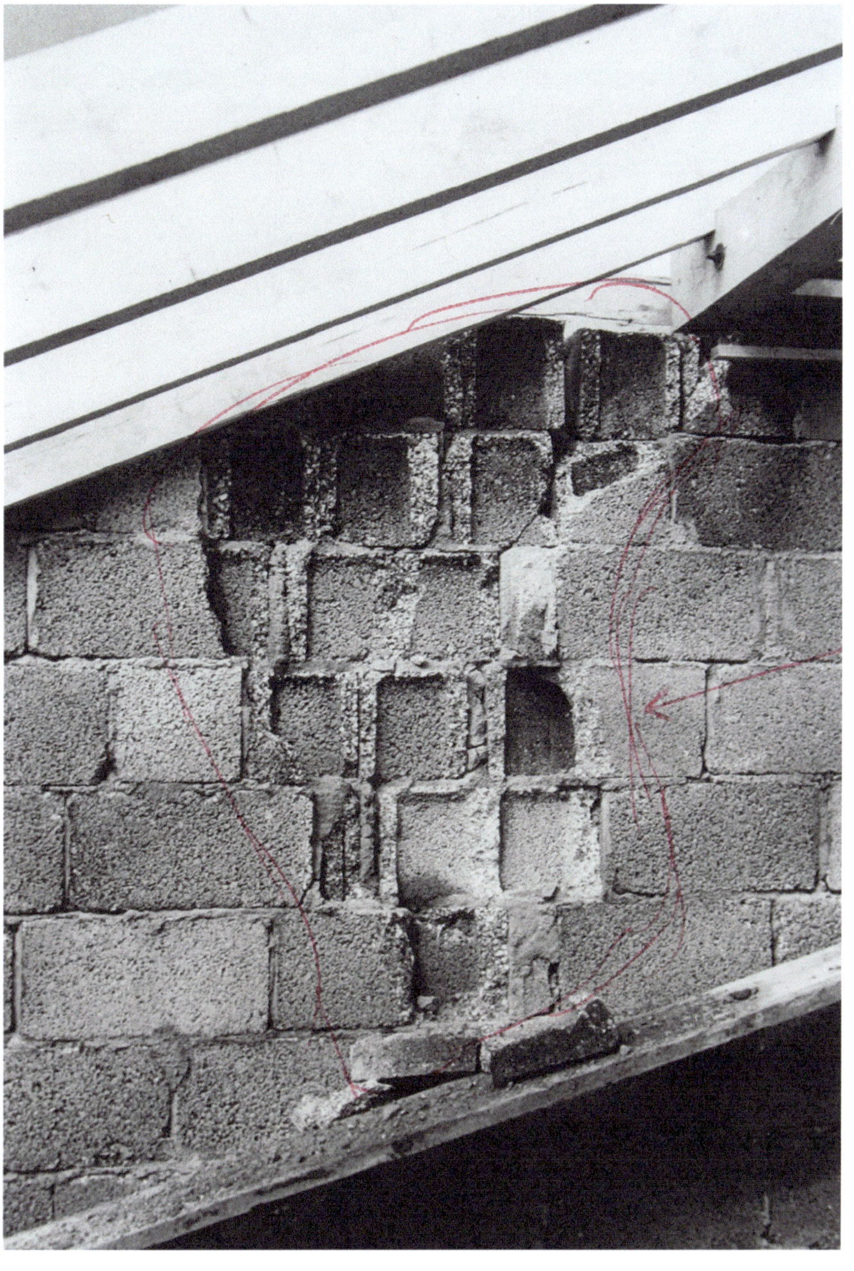

Fig. 7.7 House wall damaged by a lightning strike (*circled* and *arrow*). (Historical Collection of the Committee for Lightning Conductor Construction for the United Economic Area e. V.)

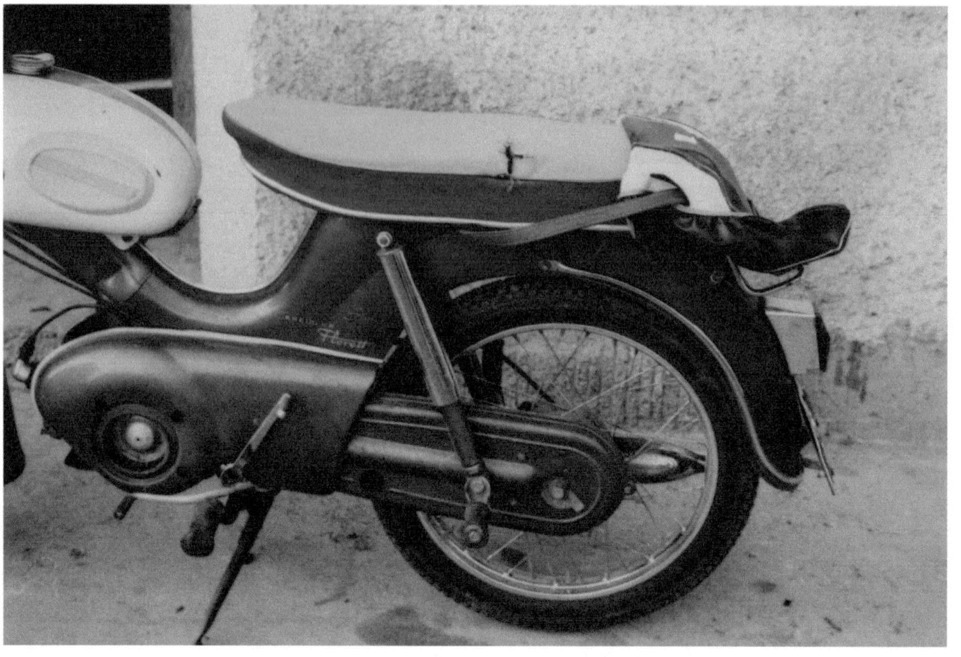

Fig. 7.8 Seat of a moped damaged by a lightning strike in the context of an accident with personal injury. (Historical Collection of the Committee for Lightning Conductor Construction for the United Economic Area e. V.)

that were characteristic of a lightning strike were found in 169 (71.9%) cases (Bingert et al. 2024).

Possible Clues from the Immediate Vicinity of the Accident Site for the Diagnosis *Lightning Strike*

- Dead mammals or birds
- Characteristic damage to trees (preferably bark)
- Burns from other plants
- Damage to houses and huts (preferably roof, wooden beams)
- Damage to the road surface or sidewalk
- Craters of up to 2 m in diameter in the ground
- Scorch marks on objects or lines
- Melting effects on metal objects
- Lichtenberg figures on objects or lawn

7.1.2 Clothing and Jewelry of the Victim

After a thorough examination of the immediate surroundings of the body, a careful inspection of the worn clothing including the contents of the pockets and, if present, the worn jewelry, a worn watch, and other items close to the body follows (Zack and Büttner 2020). Most commonly, mechanical tears and/or thermal damage to the clothing are observed. Undamaged outerwear does not necessarily mean that the garments underneath also show no findings from a lightning strike (Pollak et al. 1988). Tearing caused by the explosive pressure wave (see Chap. 4) can vary greatly in intensity and location depending on the case. However, they are described in the technical literature in all areas of worn clothing, from headgear to shoes (Figs. 7.9, 7.10, 7.11, 7.12 and 7.13) (Blumenthal 2021; Cooper et al. 2017; Krause 2004; Ohashi et al. 2001). It can also lead to the removal and ejection of worn socks and shoes (Wetli 1996).

The thermal damage to the victims' clothing is not uniform and ranges from discrete perforations to entire parts of the clothing being on fire (McCrady-Kahn and Kahn 1981; Pollak et al. 1988; Spaar 1955). Furthermore, blackish discolorations were observed at

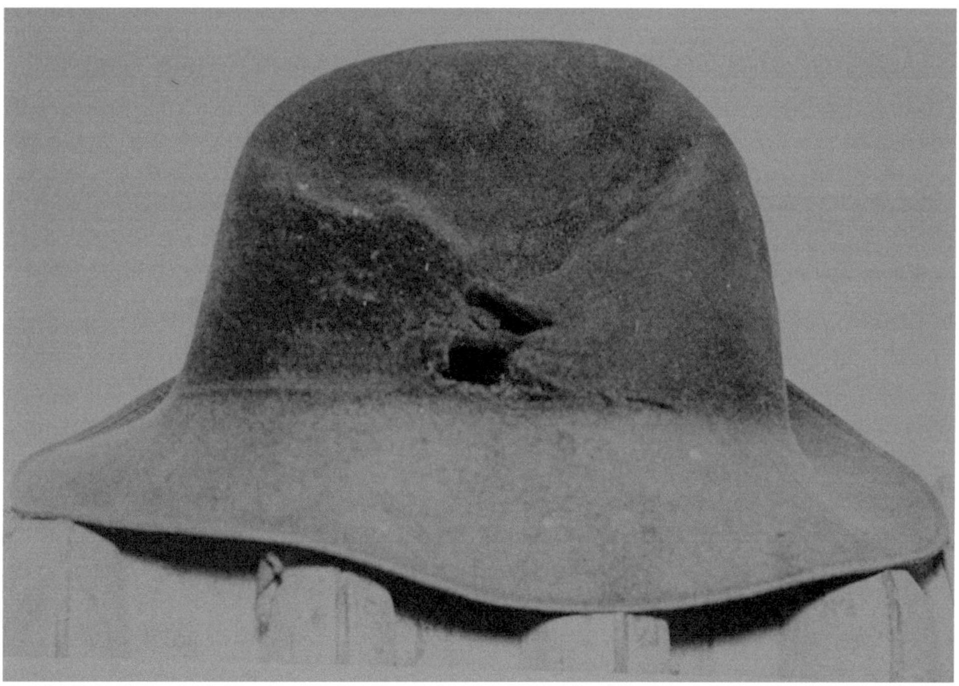

Fig. 7.9 Punctual damages of a hat after a direct hit to the head. (Historical collection of the Committee for Lightning Rod Construction for the United Economic Area e. V.)

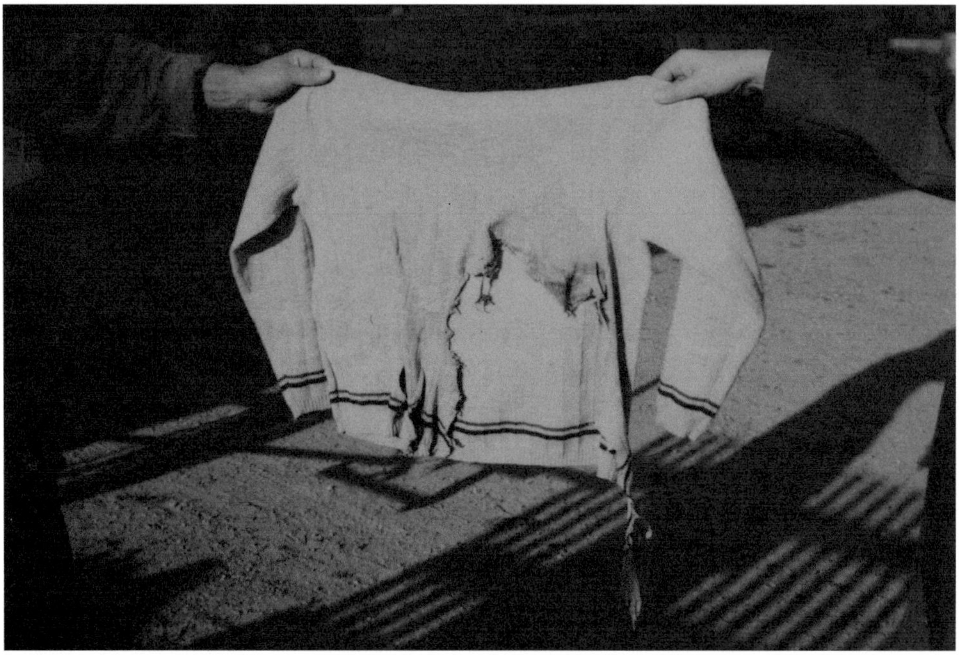

Fig. 7.10 Tears and thermal damage to a sweater. (Historical collection of the Committee for Lightning Rod Construction for the United Economic Area e. V.)

the edges of hole-like defects of a long-sleeved cotton undershirt (Fig. 7.13), in the vicinity of a zipper, and brownish-black discolorations near the metal closure of a bra (Zack et al. 2013). At torn areas of a dress shirt, macroscopically visible hardenings and curlings were described (Pollak at al. 1988). A rarity so far is the detection of a Lichtenberg figure on the outside of a leather shoe (Weimann and Prokop 1963). That even pocket contents can provide a clue to a lightning strike was demonstrated, for example, by a cigarette pack that was in the breast pocket of a torn dress shirt of a killed man and showed melting traces of the plastic cover and the foil paper of the pack (Schaidt 1977). Furthermore, melting traces were found on a coin that the victim of a lightning strike had carried in his trouser pocket (Lifschultz and Donoghue 1993b).

It was not uncommon for people who wore metal chains to suffer severe burns on the neck or for the worn jewelry to evaporate with the gaseous metal precipitating on the skin (Püschel et al. 2009; Zack et al. 2013). Furthermore, after wearing metal necklaces in lightning accidents, there have also been tattoo-like deposits of metal particles in the skin and links of the chain welded together (Jonas et al. 2002; Just et al. 2002; Pollak 2000). Metal parts of clothing, such as belt buckles, can show melting effects (Pollak

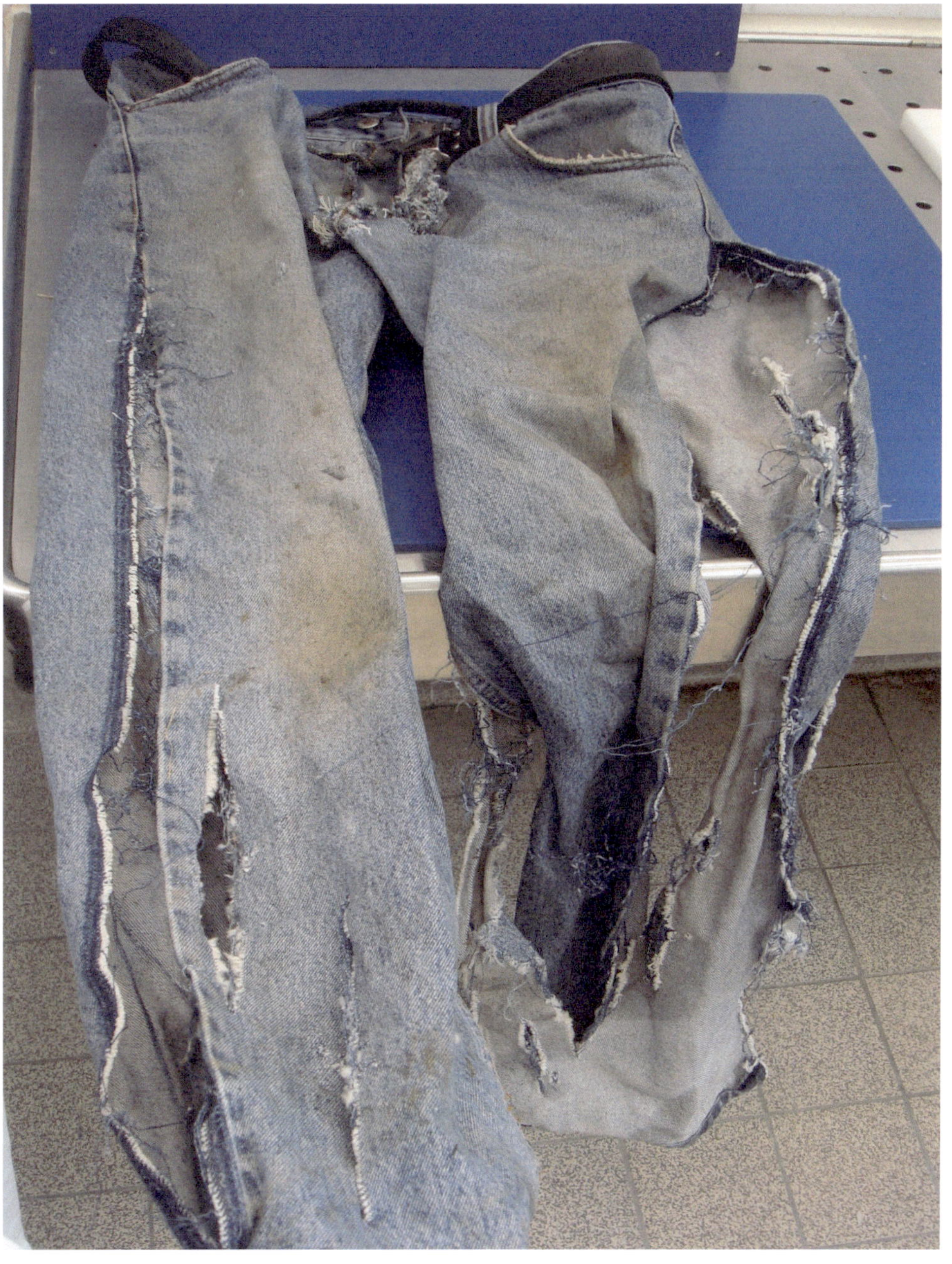

Fig. 7.11 Tears in the jeans of a deceased lightning strike victim. (Photo with kind permission: Thorsten Schwark)

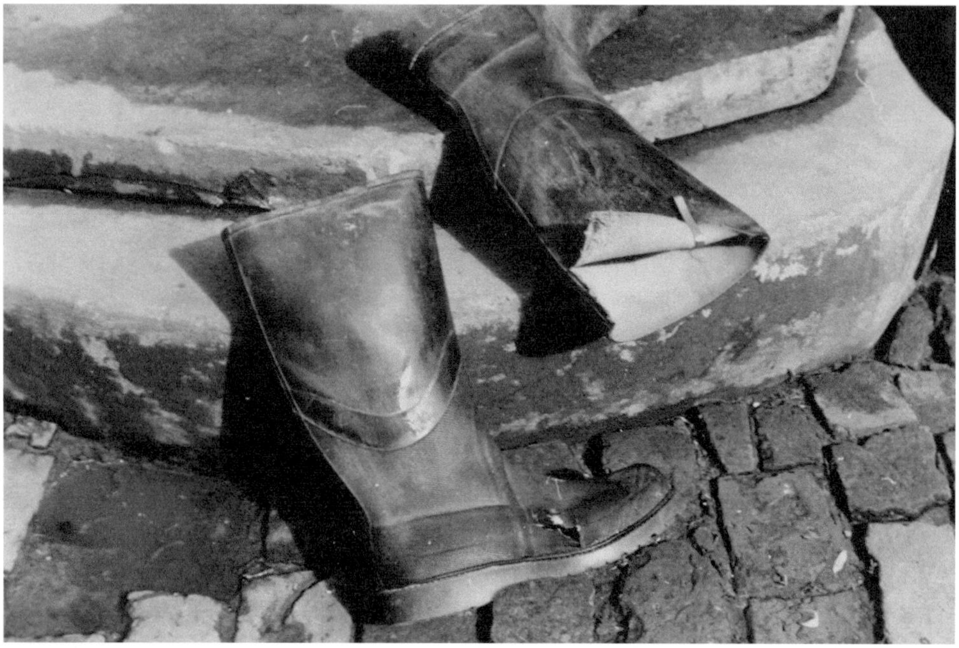

Fig. 7.12 Multiple defects in the worn rubber boots after a direct hit to the victim (Historical collection of the Committee for Lightning Rod Construction for the United Economic Area e. V.)

et al. 1988). Iron-containing objects can be magnetic after a lightning accident. For example, a victim was reported whose metal closure of the worn bra had been magnetized (Wetli 1996).

Even if a medical examiner may not have a magnifying glass in the emergency kit, it should be mentioned here that there can also be microscopic changes to clothing after a lightning strike. For example, piston-like thickenings were found at the tear sites of the fabric of damaged dress shirts, which were at least partially made of plastic (Pollak et al. 1988; Schaidt 1977). In a retrospective analysis of 223 fatal lightning strike events from Germany, findings characteristic of a lightning effect were found on the worn clothing and/or the worn jewelry in 200 (89.7%) cases (Bingert et al. 2024).

> **Note** The different energy transfers occurring in an accident due to a lightning strike often lead to tears and/or burns of the victim's worn clothing.

7.1.3 Findings on the Corpse

Only after a thorough inspection of the surroundings of the accident site and the victim's worn clothing should the careful examination of the completely undressed corpse

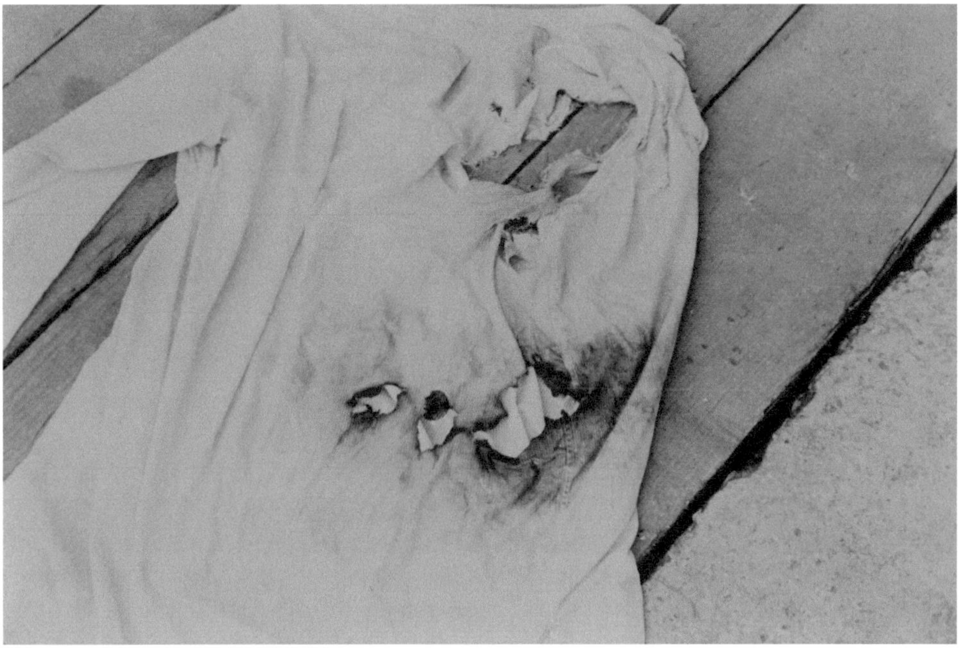

Fig. 7.13 Tears and thermal damage to a long-sleeved undershirt (Historical collection of the Committee for Lightning Rod Construction for the United Economic Area e. V.)

take place. Numerous characteristic findings can lead to the correct diagnosis, with both Lichtenberg figures and singeing of body hair being pathognomonic for death by lightning strike after excluding an accident by technical electricity (Jellinek 1903; Zack and Büttner 2020). In a retrospective analysis of 270 fatal lightning strike events from Germany, findings that were either pathognomonic or characteristic of a lightning effect were found in 259 (95.9%) cases during the external inspection of the undressed victim (Bingert et al. 2024). The following presents all findings that indicate the cause of death as lightning strike in a medical autopsy or prove it in the totality of all results.

Lichtenberg Figure

Lichtenberg figures display different patterns, which can be tree-, fern-, star-, coral- or flower-shaped (Fig. 7.14, 7.15 and 7.16). They are the result of high voltage discharges on or in insulating materials (dielectrics) and were named after the German physicist Georg Christoph Lichtenberg (1742–1799). Lichtenberg discovered this phenomenon accidentally in his laboratory when it formed as a two-dimensional pattern in the dust of a charged insulating plate. Today, it is known that Lichtenberg figures are typically caused by the rapid electrostatic discharge or redistribution of electrical charges located on the surface of insulating plates (Schroeder 1991). For the formation of Lichtenberg figures, three prerequisites are fundamentally necessary:

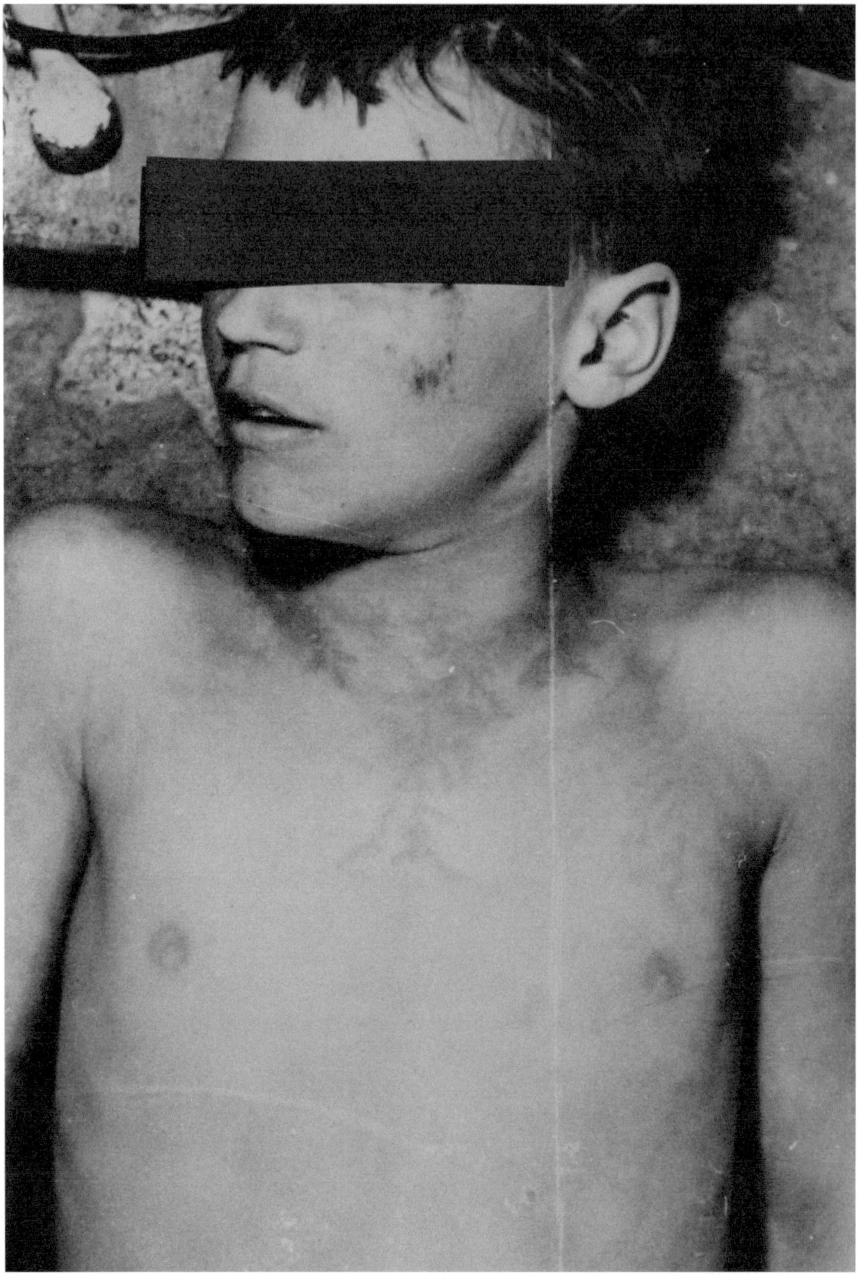

Fig. 7.14 Lichtenberg figures on the neck and upper chest region on the left of a fatally injured boy. (Historical collection of the Committee for Lightning Rod Construction for the United Economic Area e. V.)

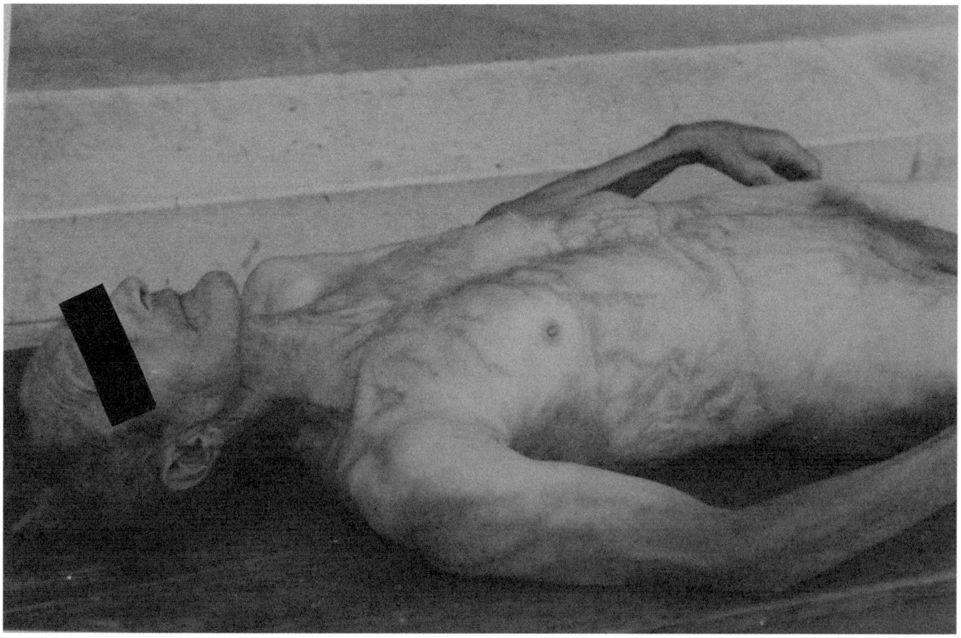

Fig. 7.15 Numerous Lichtenberg figures on the torso of a fatally injured man. (Historical collection of the Committee for Lightning Rod Construction for the United Economic Area e. V.)

- a large charge difference (e.g., during a thunderstorm between a cumulonimbus cloud and the earth),
- a discharge (e.g., by a lightning bolt), and
- a solid insulator (e.g., human skin).

Lichtenberg figures are found in victims of lightning strikes, with the exception of human skin, which acts as a solid insulator, regardless of anatomical structures such as blood vessel courses or nerves (ten Duis et al. 1987). It was a long way to this scientific realization (see Chap. 2). It is currently assumed that Lichtenberg figures are neither burns nor hemorrhages. The Lichtenberg figures on human skin are always reddish and are best explained by a transient hyperemia and dilation of the capillaries in the upper layers of the skin (Byard 2023, Pollak and Thierauf 2015; Resnik and Wetli 1996).

In the scientific literature, Lichtenberg figures are not uniformly named. In addition to the most common use of Lichtenberg figure, other terms include *"lightning figure"* (Pollak and Thierauf 2015), *"Lichtenberg flower"* (Chao 1984), *"keraunographic mark"* (Ritenour et al. 2008; ten Duis 1992; Tribble et al. 1985), *"feathering"* (feathers, plumage) (Andrews and Cooper 1992; Wetli 1996) or *"arborescent skin mark"* (Eriksson and Örnehult 1988). For the German-speaking area, it is recommended to prefer the term

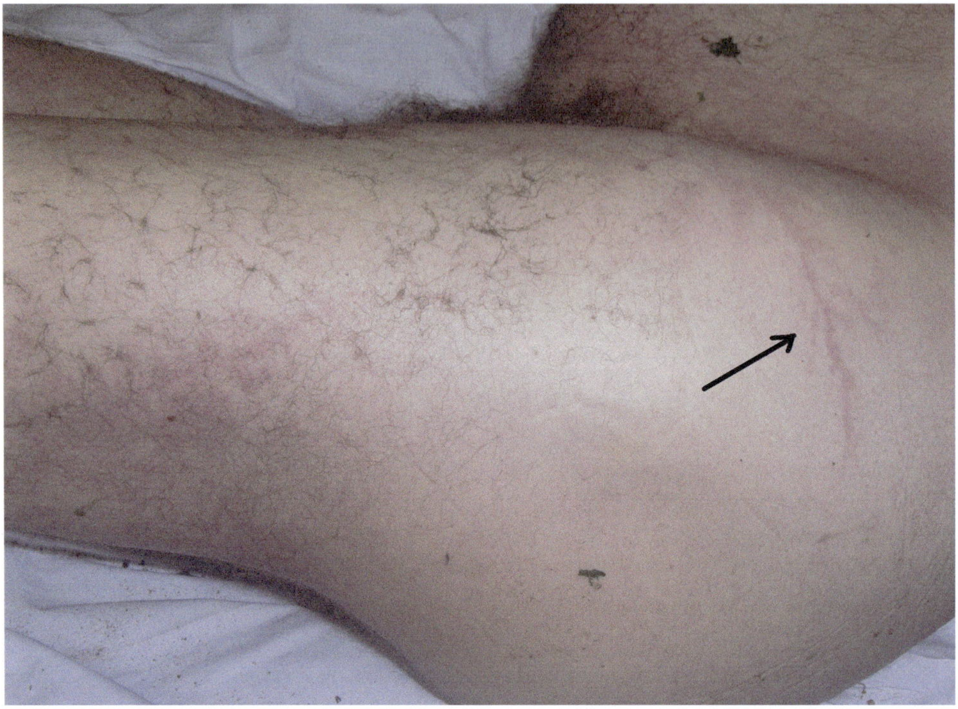

Fig. 7.16 Lichtenberg figure on the outside of the left thigh *(arrow)* in a killed victim who suffered a direct hit. (Photo courtesy: Bernd Lerche)

Lichtenberg figure over lightning figure, as a few years ago the first accident caused by technical high voltage was reported, which led to a Lichtenberg figure on the skin of a victim (Arnould and Le Floch 2011; Zack and Büttner 2016).

After their appearance, Lichtenberg figures do not remain permanently, but typically fade away over several hours until they completely disappear, both in survivors and in victims who have died as a result of the accident (Table 7.1) (Lifschultz and Donoghue 1993a; Myers et al. 1977; Perper 1976; Wetli 1996; Zack et al. 2010). The former erythema leaves no residues (Bartholome et al. 1975; ten Duis 1992; Tribble et al. 1985).

Lichtenberg figures are either extremely rare or never seen in lightning victims with dark skin. Blumenthal (2005) reported on 38 fatal lightning accidents from 1997–2000 in the South African Highveld region, of which 35 had dark skin. In the forensic examinations conducted, no Lichtenberg figure was found in any victim. Also, in the period from 2001–2022, Blumenthal, who continued to work in forensic medicine in Pretoria and was active in lightning research, found no single case of a dark-skinned victim with a Lichtenberg figure (R. Blumenthal, personal communication, January 7, 2023). In contrast, Dutta (2016) documented a Lichtenberg figure on the back of a 28-year-old dark-

Table 7.1 Duration from lightning accident to the onset of fading or complete disappearance of a Lichtenberg figure on human skin. (Own illustration)

Duration of a Lichtenberg figure on the skin		Authors
Until the onset of fading	Until complete disappearance	
n. s.	12 h	Wetli 1996
n. s.	12 h	Lifschultz and Donoghue 1993a
n. s.	19 h	Zack et al. 2010
4–6 h	n. s.	Tribble et al. 1985
17 h	24 h	Resnik and Wetli 1996
12 h	24–28 h	ten Duis et al. 1987
n. s.	24–48 h	Herold 1960
n. s.	48 h	Mutter and Langley 2019
n. s.	24–72 h	Domart 2000
n. s.	8 d	Langerhans 1862

n. s. not specified

skinned Indian woman who was struck by lightning while standing next to her bed in her house and survived the accident.

The relevance of Lichtenberg figures after a lightning accident is overestimated for forensic practice, as they can only be detected in about 17–32.5% of all victims (Eriksson and Örnehult 1988; Iranyi et al. 1962; Möhle et al. 2015; Wetli 1996; Zack and Büttner 2016). These characteristic patterns on the skin appear immediately after the lightning strike. Due to the short duration between their appearance and complete disappearance, Lichtenberg figures should be photographed as soon as possible in every case. In the investigation of lightning accidents, Lichtenberg figures have also been observed outside of human skin, for example, on a golf lawn, leather shoe, and a sidewalk slab (Cherington et al. 2003; Rakov and Uman 2006; Weimann and Prokop 1963; Zack and Büttner 2020).

The mentioned frequency of occurrence of Lichtenberg figures of 17–32.5% could be higher in practice, as it is known on the one hand that deceased victims are sometimes not fully undressed during the medical examination and the Lichtenberg figures can therefore not be recognized by the examiner. On the other hand, it is possible that in unobserved accidents the time span between the lightning strike and the medical examination is so large that Lichtenberg figures that were initially present have already disappeared by the time of the examination.

The occurrence of one or more Lichtenberg figures on the skin of a victim is, as far as an accident caused by technical electricity is not considered, proof of an accident caused by lightning. In almost all cases where the medical examination is carried out at the scene of the accident and not in a morgue, the differential diagnosis between lightning strike and technical electricity should be unproblematic.

Singeing of Hair

More than 100 years ago, Jellinek (1903) saw in the singed hair on the body of a lightning victim a *very characteristic* finding. However, to date, there is no information on the frequency of occurrence of singed hair after fatal lightning accidents for larger case numbers.

In a study of 45 deaths due to lightning strikes in Florida, Wetli (1996) found singed body hair and/or skin burns in 41 victims. Unfortunately, no differentiation was made between the two different findings.

In an evaluation of 10 fatal lightning accidents in Australia, 7 victims showed singeing of body hair, with the preferred locations being the head and pubic hair (Andrews and Cooper 1992).

In a dissertation from Mecklenburg, Schniers (2005) found singed body hair in 2 out of 4 people killed by lightning.

Lifschultz and Donoghue (1993a) found the same finding in one of 5 lightning accidents with severe consequences.

In total, singed hair was found much more frequently than Lichtenberg figures in the description of external findings after fatal lightning accidents.

The aforementioned small case numbers call for a study on the frequency of detection of singeing of body hair and Lichtenberg figures in a larger study group. A study is currently underway on a historical collection of files on lightning accidents with personal injury that occurred in the Federal Republic of Germany from 1951–1965. This case collection was organized by the former Committee for Lightning Conductor Construction in the United Economic Area e. V., subsequently passed on to the Committee for Lightning Protection and Lightning Research (ABB) of the Association for Electrical, Electronic and Information Technologies e. V. (VDE), and initially partially evaluated from an electrical engineering perspective (Harms 1956,1961). Due to the significant reduction of lethal lightning accidents in Germany over the past decades, this data collection is still extremely valuable today. After the case collection was transferred from the ABB of the VDE to the Institute of Forensic Medicine in Rostock, all lethal lightning accidents were initially evaluated as part of a medical dissertation. Of the total of 752 people who died from lightning strikes in the Federal Republic of Germany between 1951–1965, documents for 412 victims were reviewed in this collection (Bremer 2024; Schniers 2005). Of these 412 killed individuals, in 142 cases neither information nor illustrations about possible findings during an external inspection were found, if there had been any. Of the remaining 270 lethal lightning accidents, which represented 35.9% of the people killed by lightning strikes in Germany during this period, almost half, with 129 (47.8%) victims, showed singeing of body hair and significantly fewer, with 25 (9.3%) victims, showed Lichtenberg figures (Bingert et al. 2024; Bremer 2024). Based on these results, it must be assumed that singeing of body hair is significantly more common among the two diagnostic external findings (Table 7.2). The localization of this finding is dominated by the head, chest, abdominal, pubic, and leg hair (Fig. 7.17 and 7.18).

Table 7.2 Comparison of the frequencies of pathognomonic findings of hair singeing vs. Lichtenberg figures after fatal lightning accidents. (Own illustration)

Singeing of hair	Lichtenberg figure/s	Total number of cases	Authors
129	25	270	Bremer 2024
26	0	38	Blumenthal 2005
7	2	10	Andrews and Cooper 1992
1	1	5	Lifschultz and Donoghue 1993a
2	1	4	Schniers 2005

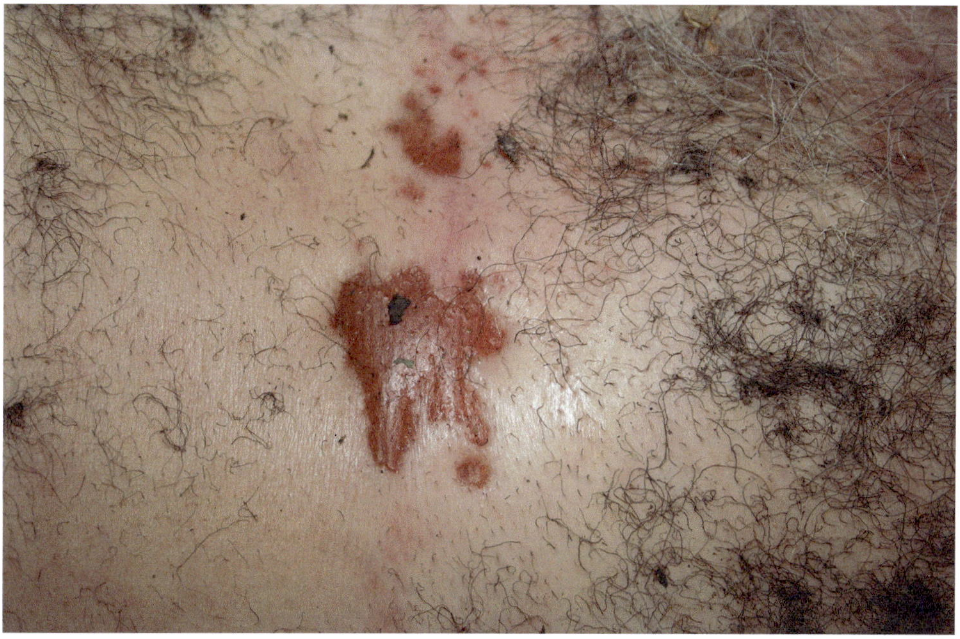

Fig. 7.17 Singed hair and skin dryness in the chest area of a fatally injured man. (Own illustration)

> **Note** Both the occurrence of singeing of body hair and Lichtenberg figures of the skin are considered, independently of each other and after excluding an accident by technical electricity, as pathognomonic for an accident by lightning strike. The occurrence of singed body hair is considerably more common.

Burns

Due to the extremely high temperatures in the lightning channel, reaching over 30,000 °C, clothing, objects, vehicles, buildings, trees, forests, fields, haystacks and much more can suddenly catch fire due to lightning strikes (Heidler and Stimper 2009; Uman 2008).

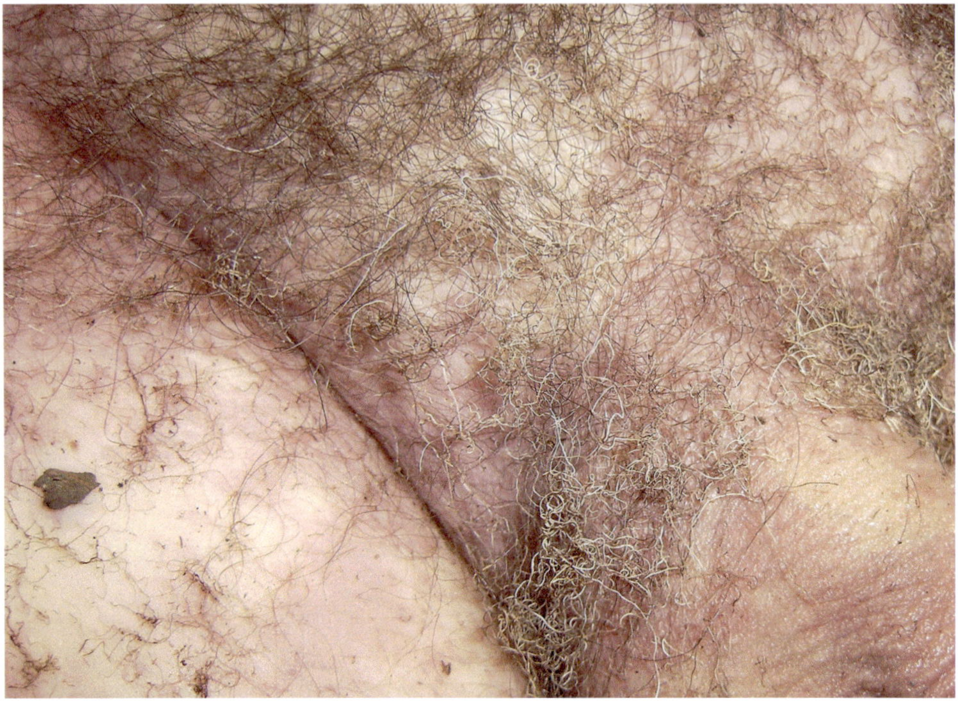

Fig. 7.18 Singed pubic hair of a fatally injured man. (Own illustration)

Immediately after lightning strikes, people have been observed with burning or still smoldering clothes (McCrady-Kahn and Kahn 1981; Spaar 1955; Tadler et al. 2017).

Burns are relatively common in lightning victims. In a study from Nebraska, 48 out of 54 severely injured people (89%) had multiple burns (Cooper 1980).

A victim of a lightning strike can have various skin burns. The following findings were most commonly observed:

- Lightning entry and exit marks ("entry/exit burns") (Fig. 7.19),
- Relatively straight and preferably vertical burns ("linear burns") (Fig. 7.20 and 7.21),
- Punctate, shotgun-like or flower-like burns (Fig. 7.21),
- Contact burns (Fig. 7.22),
- Widespread superficial erythema ("flash burns"),
- Deep burns ("full-thickness burns") (Fig. 7.19) and
- Stripe-shaped burns (Fig. 7.21) (Andrews and Cooper 1992; Arden et al. 1956; Dürwald 1986; McCrady-Kahn and Kahn 1981; O'Keefe Gatewood and Zane 2004; Pollak et al. 1988; ten Duis 1992; Weimann and Prokop 1963).

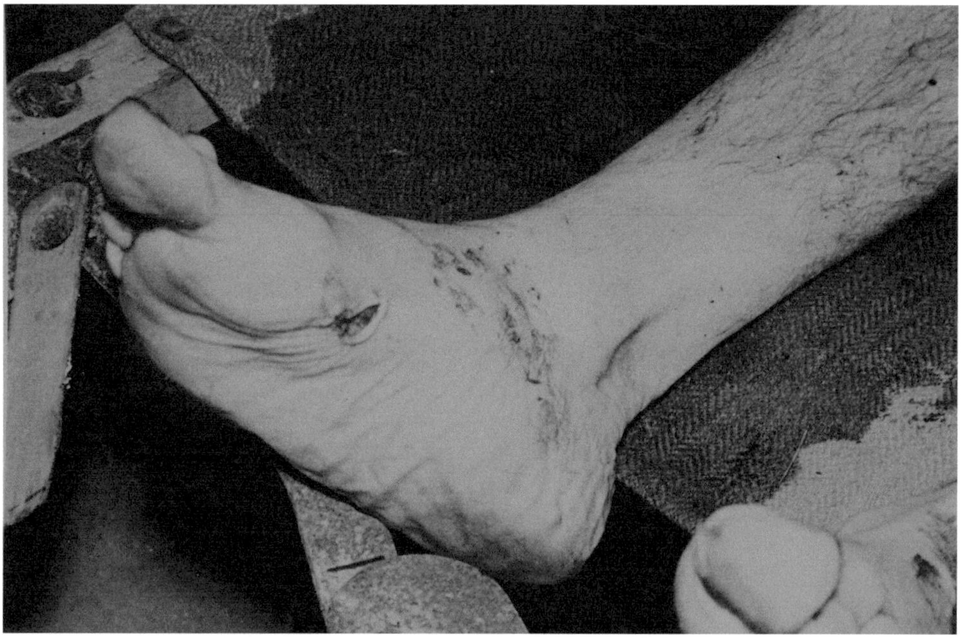

Fig. 7.19 Characteristic lightning exit mark on the inside of the right foot sole after a direct hit. (Historical Collection of the Committee for Lightning Rod Construction for the United Economic Area e. V.)

The greatest extent of burns associated with a lightning strike described in the literature so far was 70% of the body surface, with all four degrees of severity occurring (Alyan et al. 2006; Browne and Gaasch 1992; Kharoshah et al. 2023; McCrady-Kahn and Kahn 1981; Peters 1983; Pollak and Thierauf 2015; Skan 1949; Stütz et al. 2006; Ventura et al. 2017). However, 4th degree burns are extremely rare. Excluding cases with burning clothes, the reported burns of the body surface are in the range of 3.5-20% (Kilbas et al. 2008; Sleihwah et al. 2018).

▶ **Note** A large proportion of lightning victims have 1st to 3rd degree skin burns.

Lightning entry marks are, if present, found in the area of the head, neck, shoulders, upper sections of the arms or torso and often represent localized skin burns of varying depth. Cases have also been described where the entry marks consisted only of singed head hair. *Lightning exit marks*, on the other hand, are preferably found on the feet and often resemble skin injuries after accidents caused by high-voltage electrotechnology (Fig. 7.19). They, like the entry marks, show a great variety of forms (Andrews and Cooper 1992; Courtman et al. 2003; Kharoshah et al. 2023; Krauland 1951; Möhle et al.

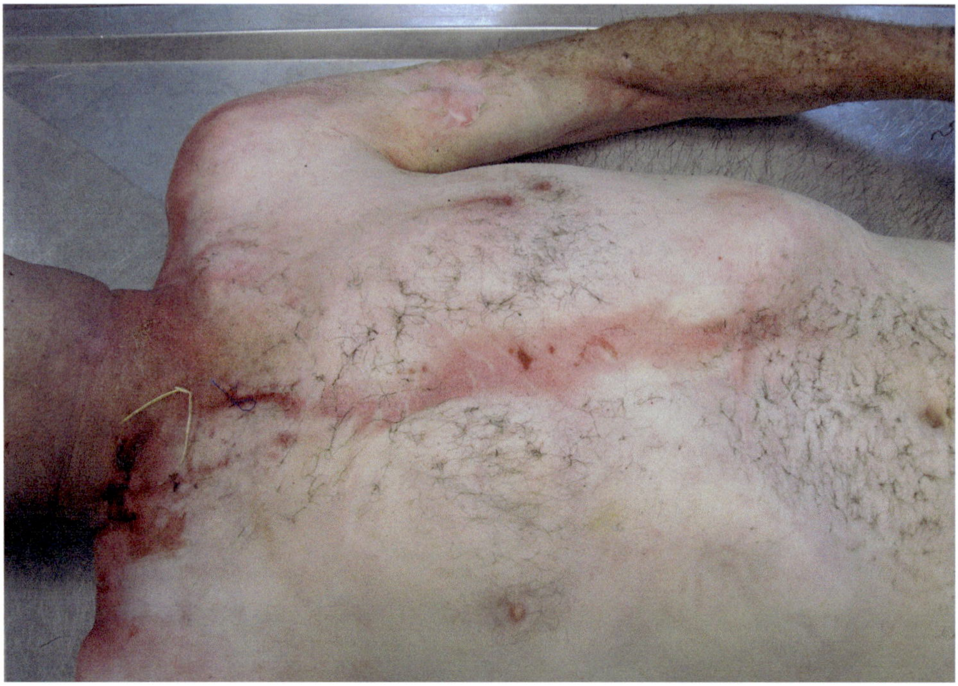

Fig. 7.20 Relatively straight, tending to be vertical burn of a killed victim after a direct hit. (Photo courtesy: Thorsten Schwark)

2015; Murty 2007; Pollak and Thierauf 2015; Pollak et al. 1988; Sellier 1975; Zack et al. 2010). The occurrence of entry and exit marks is said to be more common in victims with a dry surface than in people with soaked clothing (Blumenthal 2021).

Relatively straight-line burns are often found on the torso and tend to be vertical, corresponding to the course of the current flow on the body surface into the earth in an upright body position at the time of the lightning strike (Fig. 7.20). They are occasionally also found on the arms and legs (Alyan et al. 2006; Amy et al. 1985; Andrews and Cooper 1992; Möhle et al. 2015; Püschel et al. 2009; Zack and Büttner 2020).

Shotgun-like or flower-like burns resemble the "crocodile skin findings" in high-voltage accidents caused by technical electricity with the effect of an arc flash. Possibly, burns caused by flying hot liquids that have not evaporated at the lightning strike location are the cause (Fig. 7.21) (Blumenthal 2012; McCrady-Kahn and Kahn 1981; Zack et al. 2020).

Contact burns are usually caused by carried metal objects that are heated by the lightning strike. The location of these burns naturally depends on the position of the metal on the body at the time of the accident. In the literature, contact burns caused by necklaces, belt, trouser and shoe buckles, zippers, corset reinforcements, bra clasps, hairpins, boot irons, belt buckles, watch straps, cigarette cases, and keys have been described (Figs. 7.22 and 7.23) (Pollak 2000; Sellier 1975; own observations).

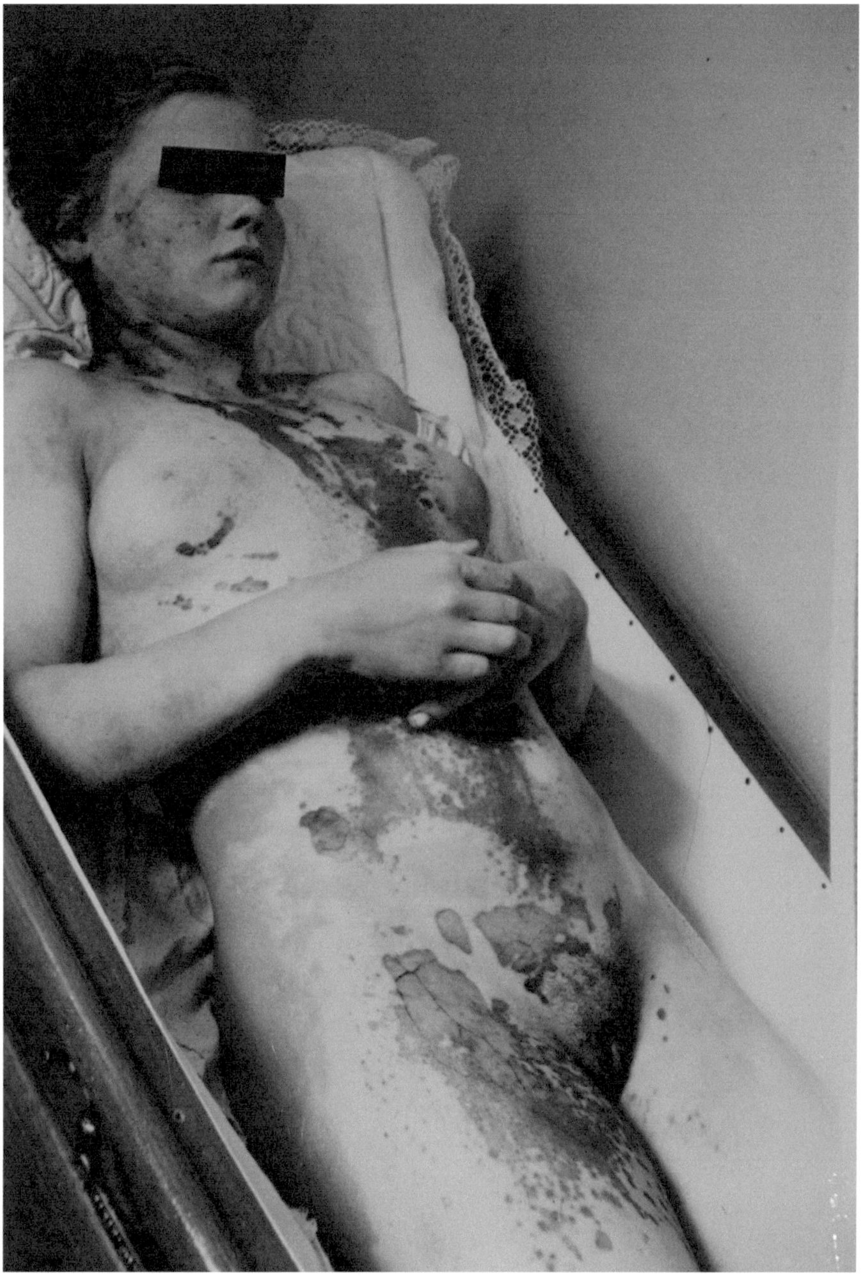

Fig. 7.21 A mixture of relatively straight (right side of the neck, upper chest region), stripe-shaped (chest and abdominal region) and shotgun-like (lower abdomen and right thigh) burns. The shotgun-like burns resemble the "Crocodile-skin findings" in high-voltage accidents caused by arc flash. (Historical Collection of the Committee for Lightning Rod Construction for the United Economic Area e. V.)

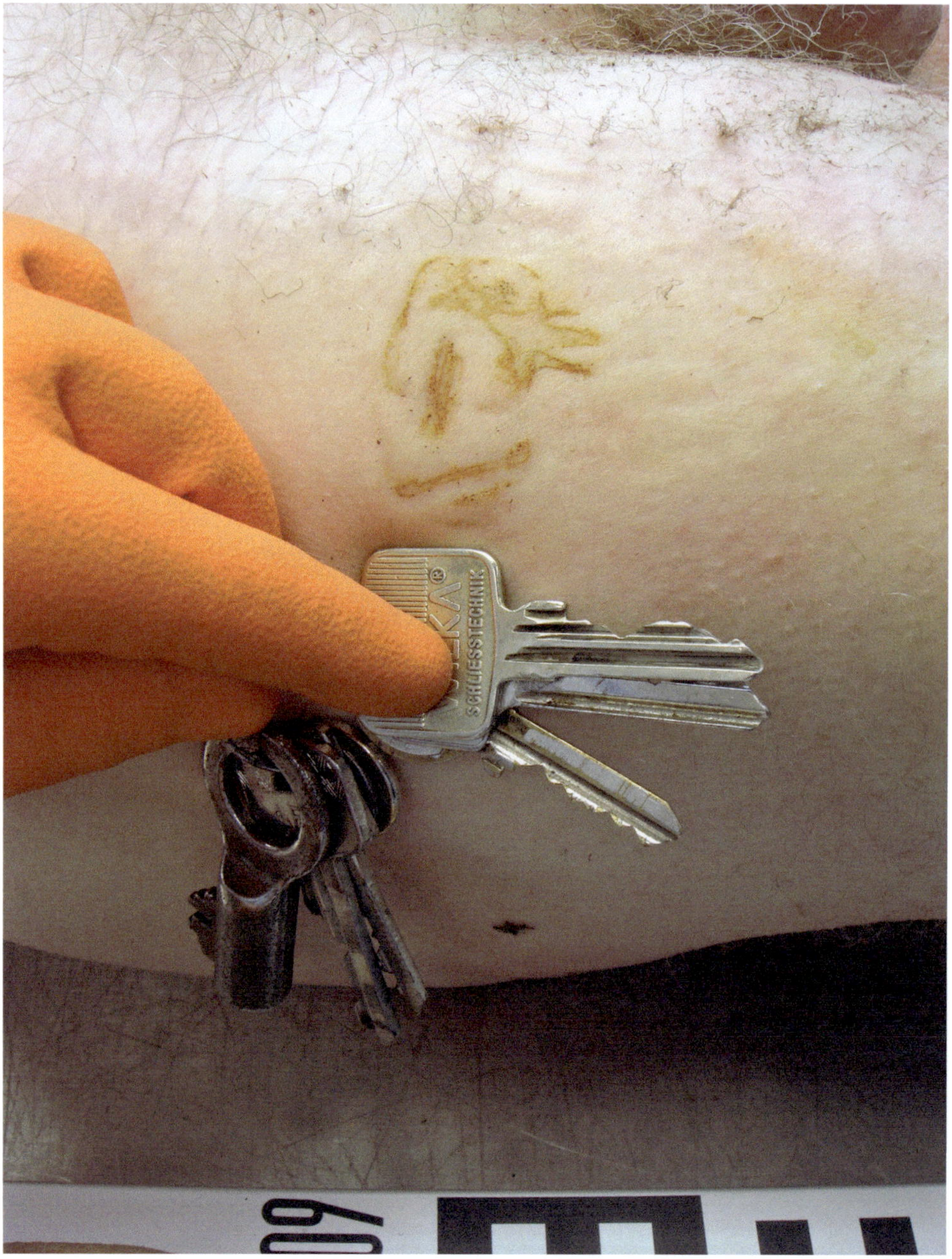

Fig. 7.22 Contact burn caused by a bunch of keys in a jeans pocket after a direct hit. (Photo courtesy: Thorsten Schwark)

Widespread superficial erythema are preferably observed on the trunk, can also have blisters in the peripheral area and heal without consequences. They are usually located in the course of the lightning current between the lightning entry and exit mark (Apanga et al. 2017; Courtman et al. 2003).

Deep burns are preferably of 3rd degree, can occur almost anywhere and in the majority of cases, depending on the location and extent of the injury, require treatment by plastic surgery (Cooper 1980; Kannan et al. 2004; Stütz et al. 2006).

> **Note** Skin burns caused by lightning are not uniform, but polymorphic.

Metallization

The energy of a cloud-to-ground lightning can heat any metal near a person so much that various findings can occur during the external inspection of an accident victim. It is possible that the metal object causes these changes especially on the skin in a solid, liquid or gaseous state. This phenomenon is also referred to as metallization in the technical literature. Whether a metal object remains solid, liquid or gaseous during a lightning strike obviously depends on its distance from the lightning channel.

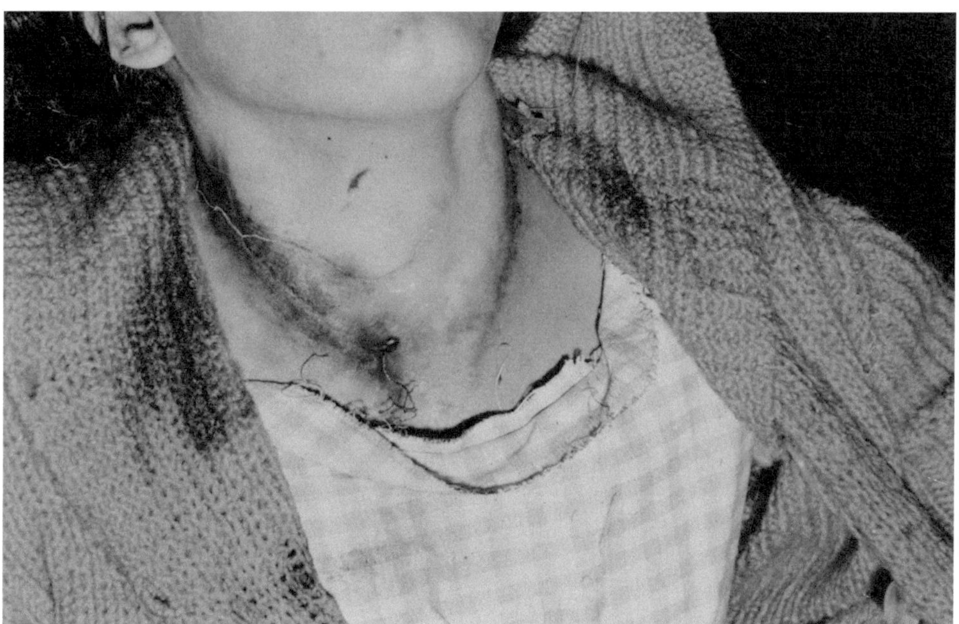

Fig. 7.23 Blackish discoloration of the neck skin and adjacent sections of the cardigan due to evaporated metal from at least one worn necklace. (Historical Collection of the Committee for Lightning Rod Construction for the United Economic Area e. V.)

Overall, three forms of metallization can occur in connection with a human lightning strike:

- a contact burn at the contact point of metallic objects (Fig. 7.22),
- a widespread deposit near evaporated metal (Fig. 7.23) and
- an intracutaneous, tattoo-like deposition of metal particles (Duppel et al. 2009; Jonas et al. 2002; Peters 1983; Pollak 2000; Pollak et al. 1988; Püschel et al. 2009; Stütz et al. 2006; Wankhede 2022; Zack et al. 2013).

Numerous case reports from the technical literature show that the neck-neck region is most frequently affected by worn metal necklaces.

Case Study

A young married couple suffered a lightning strike accident together in Mecklenburg-Vorpommern (Germany). While the man regained consciousness after a brief period of unconsciousness, the 24-year-old wife regained consciousness only after 24 hours in a clinic. Singed hair on the head, second-degree burns on the left foot, and a torn left shoe of the woman indicated an accident due to a direct hit.

While no further damage to the man was known, the female victim showed circular burns of the neck region, predominantly second degree, after wearing a necklace, a tympanic membrane perforation with subsequent temporary pancochlear inner ear deafness, and tinnitus. After conservative therapy in an ear, nose, and throat clinic, the eardrum was closed again after 3.5 months, and the accident victim showed bilateral normacusis (Just et al. 2002).

Due to a persistent tattoo-like change on the neck, the woman consulted dermatologists after her discharge from the clinic. It was then revealed that the precious metal necklace worn at the time of the accident no longer existed.

A skin biopsy performed 6 months after the accident showed the accumulation of gold particles of different sizes in the dermis, extending deep into the subcutaneous fat tissue. In semi-thin sections, histiocytes, multinucleated foreign body giant cells, and fibroblasts with ingested metal particles were detectable. In transmission electron microscopy, gold beads up to 30 μm in diameter were visible outside the cells, in the collagen matrix of the connective tissue, next to metal particles up to 5 nm in size inside lysosomes and residual bodies of phagocytes. Four different types of gold particles could be distinguished: beads, granular irregular particles, tubes, and nodular paths. In scanning electron microscopy, gold particles were detected in the connective tissue of the subcutis. Here, energy-dispersive X-ray spectroscopy elemental analysis showed strong signals of gold, silver, and copper. The detected metals were quantified by atomic absorption spectrometry as 70% gold, 21% silver, and 9% copper, which corresponded to the composition of the gold alloy of the patient's necklace. The examiners of the skin biopsy recommended the dermatologists not to attempt to remove the metal particles, as their location was too deep and too widespread (Jonas et al. 2002). ◀

Bleeding from One or Both Ears

Another finding that points to the diagnosis of *death by lightning strike* during a medical post-mortem examination is bleeding from the external ear canal after tympanic membrane rupture due to the barotrauma associated with a lightning strike (Blumenthal 2021; Cherington et al. 2001; Hunt et al. 2020). This injury can occur on one or both sides, with ruptures of both eardrums being less commonly described. The literature provides different information about the frequency of tympanic membrane ruptures in connection with a lightning strike accident, ranging from 10% (the examined collective included 5 cases) over 50% (66 cases) to over 80% (45 cases) (Cooper 1980; Lifschultz and Donoghue 1993a; Wetli 1996). Bleeding from the external ear canal will rarely suffice as a diagnostic finding in an unobserved lightning strike accident, as there are numerous other causes for bleeding from the external ear canal, such as skull base fractures, brain tumors, ear furuncles, or foreign bodies. In observed events, in addition to a tympanic membrane rupture, a skull base fracture after a severe fall may also be considered as a cause. Cherington et al. (2001) reported a case where bilateral tympanic membrane ruptures in combination with a thermal injury to a worn jogging shoe were the only findings in an unobserved death by lightning strike.

Case Study

After a 20-year-old man had gone out for a jog, he did not return from the mountains of Colorado (USA). His friends notified the police, and during the subsequent search operation the next day, the jogger was found dead on an unprotected slope. The autopsy and post-mortem examination revealed only a thermally damaged jogging shoe with melted upper material and bilateral tympanic membrane ruptures with hemotympanum. Extensive additional examinations ruled out a different cause of death. The friends reported that the sky had been cloudless when the jogger set off on a late afternoon in July. They had also not noticed any lightning or thunder afterwards, leading the investigators to diagnose death by the "bolt-from-the-blue phenomenon" (Cherington et al. 2001). ◀

Optional characteristic post-mortem findings in death by lightning strike

- Dead animals in the immediate vicinity
- Damage to objects in the immediate vicinity
- Tearing and/or thermal damage to clothing
- Thermal effects on metal objects found on the body

- Singeing of parts of body hair
- Lichtenberg figures on the skin
- Burns on the skin
- Metalization effects on or in the skin

7.1.4 Problems in Making a Diagnosis

In particular, the forensic medical literature shows that there can be numerous problems and misdiagnoses in connection with a medical examination of a corpse (Rothschild 2009; Zack et al. 2017). The causes of incorrect diagnoses are diverse. There are cases where the doctor keeps a distance of several meters from the deceased and then still issues a death certificate and bills for the "examination of the corpse," even though he has not seen essential findings (own observations).

Another error that is often detected is the doctor's sole focus on the corpse and the disregard of the immediate surroundings of the discovery site (see Sect. 7.1.1) (Blanco-Pampin et al. 1997; Schaidt 1977).

Also a common mistake that can lead to a wrong diagnosis is not undressing the deceased (see Sect. 7.1.2) (Pollak et al. 1988; Pollak 2000). Another point of criticism is the insufficient care of individual doctors during the external inspection of the deceased person. In one case from Mecklenburg-Western Pomerania, a doctor failed to recognize a suicide by electric current and documented an incorrect cause of death. The doctor performing the examination of the corpse also overlooked the electric cable, from which the suicide victim had previously removed the insulation at one end. The court-ordered autopsy, initiated at the suggestion of the police present, unequivocally provided the diagnosis *death by electric current,* which could have been made solely by external inspection (visual diagnosis) (Zack et al. 2020).

The next point, which can lead to an incorrect diagnosis of the cause of death despite consideration of the immediate surroundings, complete undressing of the deceased person, and careful examination of the corpse, is insufficient knowledge about pathognomonic or characteristic findings (Ebertz 1891; Pollak et al. 1988; Pollak 2000; Schaidt 1977).

Last but not least, even with a correctly performed medical examination of a corpse in cases with few or no findings, even after a lightning strike, there can be significant problems in making the correct diagnosis (Cherington et al. 1998; Sellier 1975).

Case Example

A married couple was caught in a storm while working in a field in Germany. While searching for a protective place, they separated. While the man ran into a nearby forest, the woman stayed in the field and lay down in a furrow. After the storm, the woman found her husband dead in the forest. The responsible professional association arranged for an autopsy of the approximately 55-year-old man, which was performed by a doctor from a pathology institute. With already existing putrefaction of the corpse, the autopsy report did not describe any skin changes that could have been attributed to a lightning strike. The cause of death was given as acute heart death, assuming that the man had overexerted himself through field work and the quick run into the forest. The professional association then refused to pay an accident pension, which the widow did not accept and sued. She claimed that her husband had died from a lightning strike. Four years after the man's death and after several instances, the deceased's clothing, which the widow had kept, was presented to a forensic doctor for assessment. The doctor found a perforation in the upper material and an incomplete detachment of the sole of the left leather shoe. Numerous tears were found on the trousers and the left sock. The expert evaluated these findings as classic signs of a lightning strike, and the case was ultimately decided in favor of the widow (Sellier 1975). ◀

Mistakes that can Lead to a Misdiagnosis during a Medical Examination of a Corpse

- Despite visiting the scene, no examination of the corpse is carried out
- Insufficient consideration of the immediate surroundings of the deceased person
- No complete undressing of the corpse
- No inspection of all body regions and body openings
- Insufficient knowledge about identified findings

7.1.5 Technical Support in Diagnosis

Both coroners and treating physicians, who are unsure based on the external findings of the injured person whether lightning strike is to be considered as the cause of the injuries, have been able to rely on the support of regional lightning detection systems for many years (see Chap. 3). If interested, any doctor and any other person can research whether cloud-to-ground lightning strikes have been registered for the relevant time period and event location. This service (Table 7.3) has so far helped to correctly classify unexplained deaths and provide concrete data on times, locations, and current strengths of the detected lightning strikes for scientific publications (Diepenseifen et al. 2009; Hunt et al. 2020; Kleiter et al. 2007; Püschel et al. 2009; Zack et al. 2013). For example, the National Lightning Detection Network of the USA was able to prove that the acute cardiac arrest of a cyclist, which occurred under a cloudless sky, was due to a lightning strike that occurred 16 km away from the associated thunderstorm cell *("bolt from the blue")* (Cherington et al. 1997).

Table 7.3 Selected examples of regional lightning detection systems. (Own representation)

Country/Region	Abbreviation	Nomenclature/Explanation
Germany	BLIDS	Lightning Information Service
Austria	ALDIS	Austrian Lightning Detection Information System
Switzerland	–	MeteoSwiss
Europe	EUCLID	European Cooperation for Lightning Detection
USA	NLDN	U.S. National Lightning Detection Network Database
Canada	CLDN	Canadian Lightning Detection Network
South Africa	SALDN	South African Lightning Detection Network

7.1.6 Diagnosis Encryption

Even though the 11th version of the International Statistical Classification of Diseases and Related Health Problems of the World Health Organization is in preparation, the encryption of the cause of death and the accident event, for example on the death certificate, is currently still according to the 10th version. For the cause of death by lightning strike, the code T75.0 (damage by lightning) and for the accident event the code X33 (victim of lightning) is provided (World Health Organisation 2022).

7.1.7 Interdisciplinary Accident Analysis

Whilein the past often involved individual scientists attempting to comprehensively investigate fatal lightning accidents (Jellinek 1903; Harms 1956; Krauland 1951; Wetli 1996), the complex topic of accident analysis has been increasingly handled by interdisciplinary teams in recent years. Not only do emergency doctors, treating physicians, and forensic pathologists cooperate, but they also seek collaboration with electrical engineers, meteorologists, statisticians, police officers, and other professional groups. The resulting broad gain in knowledge benefits all participants and thus also the coroners (Cooper et al. 2017; Hunt et al. 2020; Zack et al. 2013).

7.2 Pathophysiology of the Cause of Death

In a fatal lightning strike accident, death can occur immediately at the scene of the event or after an undefined time interval.

7.2.1 Acute Death

In cases of death by lightning strike, not all types of energy transfer are equally represented. In the case reports on fatal lightning accidents found in the professional literature, direct hits and side flashes are most common. A direct hit is easier to identify due to its often present entry and exit marks than a side flash. In both forms of energy transfer, the electrical lightning current is likely to be responsible for the immediate death at the accident site. The pathomechanisms are still not unequivocally clarified to this day. In addition to an immediate paralysis of the respiratory center, ventricular fibrillation or asystole are also mentioned. It is also discussed whether the cardiac arrest or ventricular fibrillation often observed when the emergency doctor arrives are the consequences of a generalized hypoxia due to a respiratory arrest (Andrews and Cooper 1992; Cooper 1980; Eadie 1992; Karobath et al. 1977; Pollak et al. 1988; Pollak and Thierauf 2015; Wetli 1996).

The aforementioned pathomechanisms are likely also responsible for the acute death at the accident site in the significantly less frequently reported forms of energy transfer, contact effect, wire-mediated lightning accident, and upward lightning.

Whether a received in step voltage can lead to death in humans, unlike in large mammals, is also not clarified. Reliable case reports of deaths due to an obtained step voltage are found in the professional literature only for mammals. The significantly larger distance between the legs in large animal species leads to a considerably higher risk of being fatally injured by the received step voltage in a lightning accident. Here too, the current flow over the heart with subsequent ventricular fibrillation or asystole is most likely responsible for the simultaneous death of several animals (Badagliacca et al. 2017; Carte et al. 2002; Rakov and Uman 2006; Stoff et al. 2020).

However, a person can also die in the context of a lightning accident independently of the electrical energy. In these cases, deaths caused by both thermal and mechanical energy are found at the accident site.

For all lightning accidents where there has not been a fire at the accident site, the intensity and extent of skin burns observed on the victims' body surface are not sufficient to cause a person's death (Zack and Büttner 2020). However, lightning accidents that lead to an open fire have repeatedly caused the death of individuals (Holle 2010; Ventura et al. 2017). In these cases, death can occur either through smoke inhalation poisoning or through local heat damage to the skin and underlying tissues and organs in the sense of an acute burn death. In the case of death by smoke inhalation poisoning, the inhalation of carbon monoxide is paramount, which, due to its significantly higher affinity for hemoglobin, displaces oxygen from its bonds with the red blood pigment and thus causes death through "internal" suffocation.

The application of significant mechanical energy is another form of energy transfer in a lightning accident that can lead to immediate death at the scene. The explosive expansion of the highly heated air in the lightning channel and the subsequent pressure wave can throw individuals against hard objects or surfaces, or movable objects can hit a person's body. In these cases, intracranial hemorrhages or brain contusions are usually the injuries leading to death (Blumenthal 2021; Bremer 2024).

Furthermore, it should be mentioned in the context of the pathophysiology of the cause of death that acute deaths in individuals who show no externally visible injuries are attributed to the magnetic field occurring in the immediate vicinity of a discharge phase. In such cases, ventricular fibrillation or asystole are held responsible for the onset of lethal exitus (Cherington et al. 1998; Heidler and Stimper 2009).

A case of death in which there was supposed to have been a complete destruction of the body immediately after a lightning strike, as claimed in a advanced education article without an accompanying case study (Bartsch 2013), has not been found in the medical literature so far.

Common Pathophysiological Mechanisms in Acute Death by Lightning Strike

- Ventricular fibrillation or asystole
- Central respiratory paralysis
- Acute burn death
- Acute smoke inhalation poisoning
- Intracranial hemorrhage
- Brain contusion

7.2.2 Death After a Time Interval

For the victims of a lethal lightning strike accident who did not die immediately, the interval between the time of the accident and the time of death varies (Table 7.4). An evaluation of 30 case reports from the medical literature, which provided specific information about this time interval, shows a range from 10.5 hours to 6 years. In 24 out of 30 cases (80%), death occurred within the first two weeks after the accident. In a case of death from a glioblastoma after a lightning strike suffered 14 months earlier, the investigators affirmed the causal connection (Cherington et al. 1994). However, this assessment was not uncontested (Andrews and Reisner 2017).

As is known from numerous epidemiological studies (see Sect. 7.4), in this evaluation too, the male gender was most frequently affected with 26 cases (86.7%). The age of the deceased persons ranged from 8–79 years.

For diseases or injuries indirectly leading to death, lightning traumatic myocardial necrosis/acute myocardial infarction/ intramyocardial bleeding (11 times) and/or hypoxic brain damage (9 times) were predominantly reported, followed by pneumonia(5 times), multiple organ failure (4 times), intramyocardial bleeding in the sense of a contusio cordis (3 times) and/or intracranial bleeding (3 times) (Aydin et al. 2018; Blumenthal

Table 7.4 Time interval and cause of death after initially surviving a lightning strike accident. (Own representation)

No	Time Interval	Age (Years)	Gender	Cause of Death	Authors
1	10.5 h	19	m	Intramyocardial Hemorrhage	Wetli 1996
2	12 h	9	m	Aspiration Pneumonia and Lightning Traumatic Myocardial Necrosis	Hanson and McIlwraith 1973
3	20 h	21	m	Acute Myocardial Infarction	Aydin et al. 2018
4	24 h	44	m	Bronchopneumonia due to Burns of 3rd Degree and Intracranial Hemorrhages	Spaar 1955
5	24 h	24	f	Disseminated Intravascular Coagulation and Lightning Traumatic Myocardial Necrosis	Ekoe et al. 1985
6	27 h	36	m	Intramyocardial Hemorrhage	Wetli 1996
7	36 h	26	m	Hypoxia, Metabolic Acidosis, Rhabdomyolysis and Abdominal Compartment Syndrome	Geary et al. 2015
8	3 days	15	m	Hypoxic brain damage after Ventricular fibrillation in subepicardial bleeding in the vicinity of a coronary artery	Wetli 1996
9	3 days	29	m	Pneumonia due to brain damage	Krauland 1951
10	3 days	8	m	Hypoxic brain damage and acute Myocardial infarction	Harwood et al. 1978
11	3 days	57	m	Hypoxic brain damage after Cardiac arrest	Cherington et al. 1995
12	4 days	50	f	Hypoxic brain damage and Multiple organ failure	Zack et al. 2013
13	4 days	55	m	Hypoxic brain damage, acute Myocardial infarction and acute Renal failure	Whitcomb et al. 2002
14	4 days	35	m	Aspiration pneumonia and Multiple organ failure	Möhle et al. 2015
15	5 days	44	m	Hypoxic brain damage and acute Myocardial infarction	Karadas et al. 2013
16	5 days	27	m	Hypoxic brain damage and lightning-traumatic myocardial necrosis	Zack et al. 1997
17	7 days	9	m	Hypoxic brain damage and acute Myocardial infarction	Kotagel et al. 1982

(continued)

Table 7.4 (continued)

No	Time Interval	Age (Years)	Gender	Cause of Death	Authors
18	8 days	20	m	Multi-organ failure	Gruhn et al. 2016
19	9 days	15	m	Hypoxic brain damage and lightning-traumatic myocardial necrosis	Hanson and McIlwraith 1973
20	10 days	15	m	Multi-organ failure after lightning-traumatic myocardial necrosis	Kravitz et al. 1977
21	10 days	10	f	Intramyocardial hemorrhage	Blumenthal 2021
22	11 days	17	m	Hypoxic brain damage after Cardiac arrest	Schwab et al. 1989
23	11 days	22	m	Acute Respiratory Distress Syndrome after gastric perforation	Kilbas et al. 2008
24	13 days	20	m	Subarachnoid hemorrhage and intracerebral bleeding	Mann et al. 1983
25	18 days	32	m	Hypoxic brain damage after cardiac arrest	Cherington et al. 1998
26	29 days	79	m	Esophageal perforation	Figgis and Alvarez 2012
27	84 days	24	m	Bronchopneumonia after Subarachnoid hemorrhage	Forster et al. 2013
28	4 months	22	m	Myelopathy	Davidson and Deck 1988
29	14 months	64	f	Glioblastoma	Cherington et al. 1994
30	6 years	n. s.	n. s.	Hypoxic brain damage	Wetli 1996

m male, f female, n. s. not specified

2021; Cherington et al. 1994, 1995, 1998; Davidson and Deck 1988; Figgis and Alvarez 2012; Forster et al. 2013; Gruhn et al. 2016; Hanson and McIlwraith 1973; Harwood et al. 1978; Karadas et al. 2013; Kotagel et al. 1982; Krauland 1951; Kravitz et al. 1977; Mann et al. 1983; Möhle et al. 2015; Schwab et al. 1989; Spaar 1955; Wetli 1996; Zack et al. 1997, 2013). All other diagnoses, such as rhabdomyolysis, compartment syndrome, acute kidney failure or acute respiratory insufficiency due to damage to the alveolocapillary membrane after gastric perforation were only mentioned in individual cases as the cause of death from a lightning strike (Geary et al. 2015; Kilbas et al. 2008; Whitcomb et al. 2002).

> **Note** In the case of acute death, a person is most likely to die from ventricular fibrillation, asystole or central respiratory paralysis. In the event of death after a time interval, hypoxic brain damage and/or acute lightning traumatic myocardial necrosis are often responsible for the death.

7.3 Autopsy

In contrast to other types of accidents, the correct cause of death after a lightning strike is much less often determined by an autopsy than by a thorough external post-mortem examination of the body (see Sect. 7.1). This is particularly due to the fact that the most common findings leading to a correct diagnosis after an accident due to a lightning strike are not detectable by an internal, but by a careful external examination of the body (Blumenthal 2021; Zack and Büttner 2020). However, there have also been case reports where the autopsy provided the decisive findings for the clarification of a mysterious death case, after no indications of death by lightning strike were noticed at the external post-mortem examination of the body of the deceased (Cherington et al. 2001; Zack et al. 1997).

The results of an autopsy can also be misinterpreted if the examiners have no or insufficient knowledge about characteristic findings of the victim after a lightning strike. Thus, Ebertz (1891) described a lethal lightning accident from Baden-Württemberg (Germany), in which the autopsy, despite a detected Lichtenberg figure on the right rib arch of the deceased, had come to the conclusion that the autopsy had hardly provided an explanation for the acute death. Over 80 years later, after the specialist knowledge about characteristic findings after a lightning accident of a human had been significantly increased compared to 1891, Sellier (1975) reported about an autopsy, where the diagnostic leading damages on the worn clothing of the victim had been disregarded. The examiners came to the misdiagnosis "acute cardiac death", which was only corrected by a re-evaluation of the death case by an experienced or well-read doctor (see Sect. 7.1.4).

An autopsy regularly involves an external and internal inspection. To avoid repetitions, all findings that can be obtained during an external inspection at an autopsy are referred to the section on external post-mortem examination (see Sect. 7.1).

The following presents selected, preferably frequent findings that have been determined during an internal post-mortem examination, including histological examinations, in victims of a lightning strike.

Ears

A uni- or bilateral tympanic membrane rupture is one of the most common injuries after a lightning strike and is caused by a barotrauma (Blumenthal 2021; Murty 2009). In a case of death in the USA, a bilateral tympanic membrane rupture with bleeding into the tympanic cavities was the only finding leading to the correct diagnosis at the autopsy of a

22-year-old man who had died unobserved while jogging in the mountains (Cherington et al. 2001) (see Sect. 7.1.3).

In a retrospective analysis of 45 people who died after lightning accidents in the USA, information about examinations of the middle ear region was only found in 21 cases. In these, ruptures of the tympanic membrane were found in 17 (81%) cases, which were unilateral in 10 cases and bilateral in 7 cases (Wetli 1996).

Compared to the frequently observed tympanic membrane ruptures after a lightning accident, dislocations of the ossicles have rarely been described (Krauland 1951).

Skull and Brain

In addition to cerebral edema, which is also observed in many other causes of death and is considered uncharacteristic, hemorrhages were the most common pathological findings in the skull-brain region in victims of lightning strikes. Subarachnoid hemorrhages dominated, occurring in cases with observed fall events as well as without indications of a severe traumatic brain injury (Kleinschmidt-DeMasters 1995; Oruc et al. 2023). When subarachnoid hemorrhages were associated with significant blunt force trauma to the head, further intracranial hemorrhages were sometimes observed, which had different locations (subdural, epidural) (Spaar 1955; Strasser et al. 1977). In connection with a ruptured eardrum, there was also bleeding into the petrous bone (Hunt et al. 2020). In addition to the extracerebral hemorrhages, the occurrence of intracerebral hemorrhages was repeatedly described. Hemorrhages in the basal ganglia with rupture into the ventricular system were each found in cases of death that had a time interval of 24 hours or 13 days between the accident and the time of death (Jellinek 1903; Mann et al. 1983; Spaar 1955). Furthermore, pinpoint cortical hemorrhages were found after a 4-day survival time of a 35-year-old man who had been thrown several meters through the air at the accident site (Möhle et al. 2015). This finding was most likely caused by a brain contusion. In rare cases, victims with intracranial hemorrhages also had a skull fracture (Mann et al. 1983; Spaar 1955).

The interpretation of the causes of all hemorrhages occurring in connection with a lightning accident depends on knowledge of the discovery situation and the reconstruction of the accident.

Different macroscopic findings were extremely rare in the skull-brain region of lightning victims. For example, a pons infarction was observed in a 79-year-old man after a survival time of 15 days, and the development of a glioblastoma in a 64-year-old woman who had survived her accident for 14 months (Cherington et al. 1994; Eriksson and Örnehult 1988). A causal connection between the accident and the glioblastoma was critically viewed by other scientists (Andrews and Reisner 2017).

In the histological examinations of the brain, a variety of and little characteristic tissue changes have been described so far. The findings range from tissue severances, vessel ruptures, hemorrhages of different locations, edemas, tortuosities of brain vessels, swellings of the endothelia, perivascular halo formations, palisade-like arrangements of endothelial cell nuclei to nerve cell damage and other changes in the anatomical structures (Jellinek

1903; Kleinschmidt-DeMasters 1995; Peters 1956; Spaar 1955). The interpretation of the pathogenesis of numerous histological findings in cases of death after performed resuscitation measures, a time interval from the accident to the time of death, or a longer corpse lying time until the autopsy is particularly problematic (Peters 1956).

Due to the significant decrease in the number of annual deaths from lightning strikes in developed countries and the often much too low autopsy rates of these states, a relevant increase in expert knowledge in this field of lightning research is not necessarily to be expected in the near future (Cooper and Holle 2019).

Case Study

A 35-year-old farm worker sought shelter during a thunderstorm in North Rhine-Westphalia (Germany) on an afternoon of a harvest day in 1952 in a beet pile. The next morning, he was found dead in a sitting position. During an autopsy of the unobserved accident at a forensic institute, tears were found in the man's cap, jacket, and shirt. Upon external inspection of the body surface, both singeing of the head hair in the left temple region and superficial skin burns from the left temple region to the left cheek as well as from the jugular fossa to the right thigh were observed. Upon internal inspection, no pathological findings were found, except for the brain. After consulting a neuropathologist, changes in the brain surface in the form of clay-like consistency, wrinkling, and subarachnoid hemorrhage were found after formalin fixation of the brain, each corresponding to the location of the scorched head hair. Histological examinations showed dilation of the meningeal blood vessels, palisade-like arrangement of endothelial cell nuclei, perivascular halo formations, hemorrhages, and spongy tissue loosening in the subcortical white matter (Peters 1956). ◄

Heart

Among the internal organs with pathological findings after a lightning accident, the heart is often involved. There is no uniformity of damage. In addition to hemorrhages, acute lightning-traumaticmyocardial necroses without pathological changes of the coronary arteries and thermally damaged areas are described. The observed bleedings can occur subepicardially, intramyocardially, or subendocardially (Fig. 7.24) (Blumenthal 2021; Möhle et al. 2015; Wetli 1996; Zack et al. 1997). The intensities and locations of the cardiac hemorrhages suggest in many cases, in relation to resuscitation-related injuries, much more a contusio cordis or a barotrauma as triggers. Ischemic causes were denied in the case reports (Blumenthal 2021; Wetli 1996; Zack et al. 1997). A 15-year-old boy, who had not been resuscitated at the scene of the accident, showed a tear of the pericardium and 100 ml of bloody fluid in the pericardial sac at autopsy (Wetli 1996).

In individuals who have survived a lightning strike for a certain period of time, infarct-typical histological findings can be found. The changes in the tissue depend on the survival time. For example, extensive myocardial necroses with hemorrhages, monogranulocytic infiltration, and contraction bands were observed in an interval of 4 and

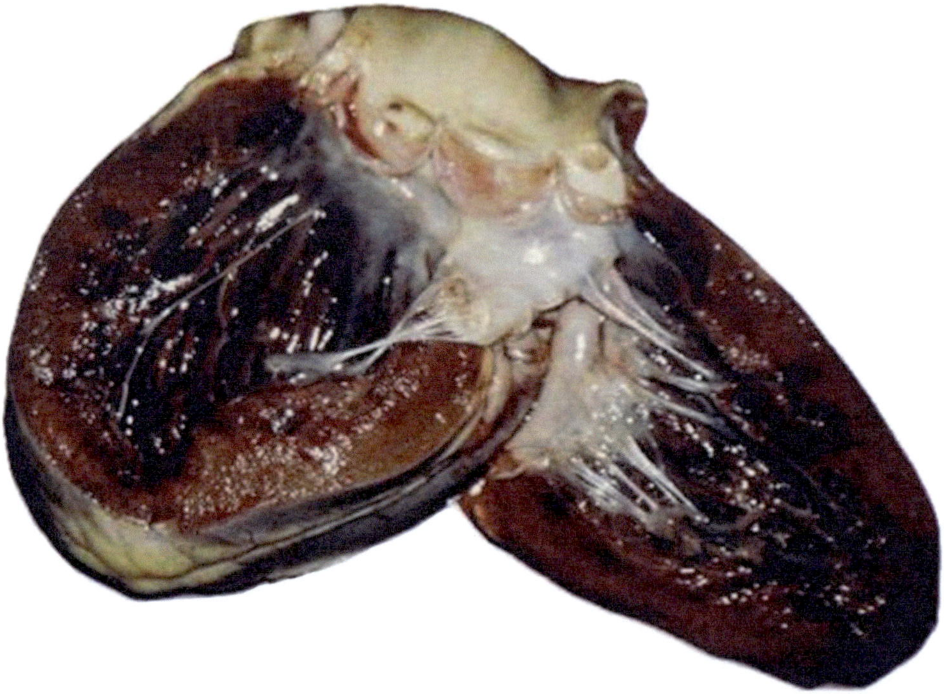

Fig. 7.24 Subendocardial and intramyocardial hemorrhages in a 27-year-old victim of an accident by side flash, who died 5 days after the accident. (Own illustration)

5 days between the lightning accident and death (Fig. 7.25, 7.26, 7.27 and 7.28) (Dettmeyer 2018; Möhle et al. 2015; Zack et al. 1997). In a survival time of 10 days, the heart of a 15-year-old boy showed numerous fibroblasts in the interstitium in addition to myolysis (Kravitz et al. 1977). The myocardium of a 53-year-old man who died at the scene of the accident showed an abnormal arrangement and fragmentation of the myocytes in the histologicalexamination (Ventura et al. 2017). In another case, a wave-like arrangement of the myocytes was observed after a lightning strike (Janssen 1984).

The pathophysiological mechanism responsible for the occurrence of an acute myocardial infarction after a lightning strike is most likely the lack of blood flow to the coronary arteries during the time of asystole or ventricular fibrillation until the onset of sufficient resuscitation measures. Even though the diagnosis of *acute myocardial infarction* has been mentioned in numerous publications in the medical literature, it is not pathophysiologically certain to be an *infarction,* as an ischemic cause of this lightning strike sequel is not proven. Therefore, with the current state of science, one should rather speak of a *lightning-traumatic necrosis* than of a myocardial infarction (R. B. Dettmeyer, personal communication, April 6, 2023; Pschyrembel 2020).

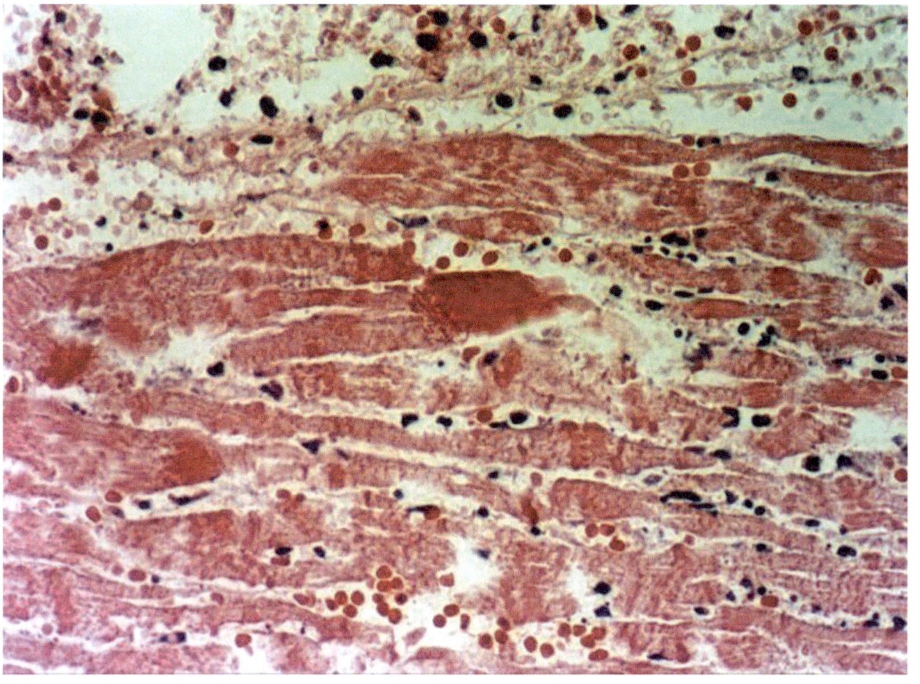

Fig. 7.25 Myocardial infarction-like findings 5 days after a lightning strike with eosinophilia of individual myocytes and inflammatory-resorptive reaction to the myolysis (HE, 224:1). (Own illustration)

Lungs and Mediastinum

Pathological findings of the respiratory tract or the mediastinum in fatally injured lightning victims have so far been relatively rarely described. A detected pulmonary edema is uncharacteristic and can be explained by the ventricular fibrillation often observed in the dying phase. The lungs and the mediastinum can be particularly damaged by the barotrauma often occurring in a lightning accident. Macroscopically, visible lung hemorrhages and histologically detectable alveolar wall ruptures are found (Ebertz 1891; Krauland 1951; Murty 2009). In rare cases, a pneumomediastinum can also occur after a lightning accident (Blumenthal and Saayman 2017).

Kidneys

If a lightning strike is temporarily survived, the kidneys can develop acute tubularnecroses of the ischemic type due to insufficient blood flow or acute tissue necrosis of the toxic type at the same location due to the release of myoglobin in necroses of the skeletal muscles, which can lead to acute kidney failure (Crush syndrome) and thus also to death (Blumenthal 2021; Whitcomb et al. 2002).

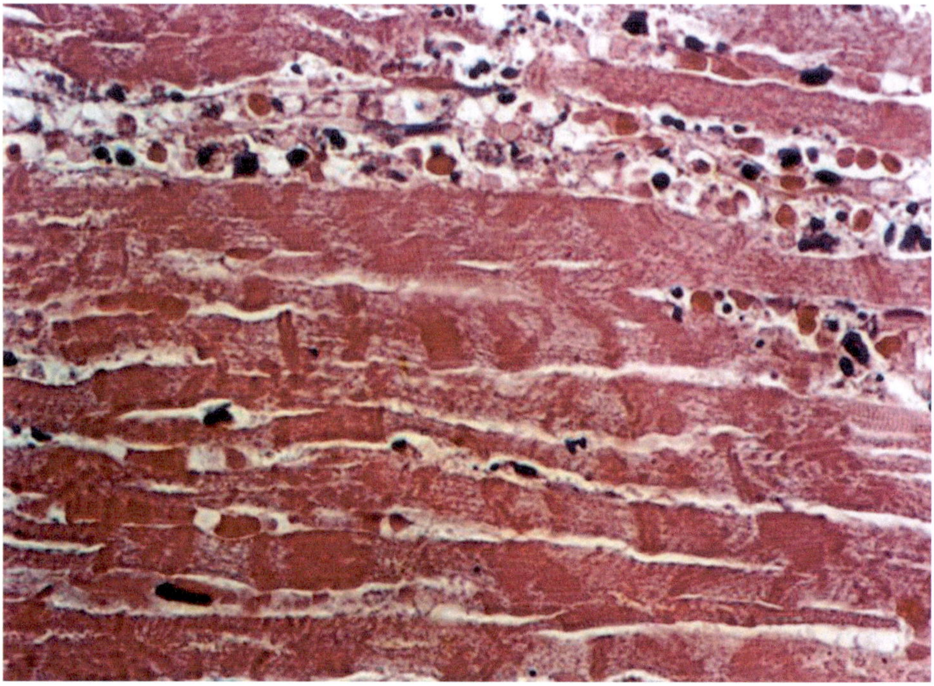

Fig. 7.26 Myocardial infarction-like findings 5 days after a lightning strike with contraction bands and mixed-cellular resorptive reaction of the myolysis (HE, 224:1). (Own illustration)

Aorta

Wetli (1996) found pathological findings on the aorta in 3 out of 45 fatal accidents caused by lightning strikes. This resulted in tears of the tunica media and only histologically detectable detachments of the tunica intima from the tunica media.

Skeletal Muscles

After a lightning accident by side flash, a 27-year-old man who died 5 days after the event due to hypoxic brain damage after ventricular fibrillation showed no externally visible injuries at the autopsy. After preparation of the skin in the area of the thorax, the victim showed extensive, almost whitish coagulations of the left chest muscles (Fig. 7.29). Histologically, extensive areactive necroses were found (Fig. 7.30) (Zack and Büttner 2020).

> **Note** Even though the diagnosis *death by lightning strike* is most often made by a careful external post-mortem examination of the body, there are accidents that can only be clarified by an autopsy.

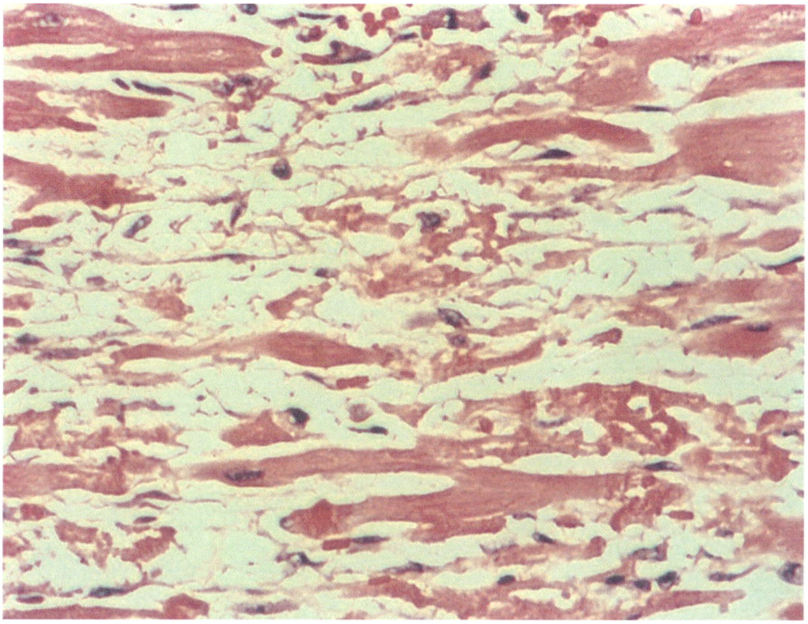

Fig. 7.27 Necrosis of the myocytes with destruction of the myocardial structures 5 days after a lightning strike (HE, 224:1). (Own illustration)

Skin

Since the macroscopic findings of the skin that a victim can exhibit after a lightning accident have already been described during the external post-mortem examination (see Sect. 7.1.3), only the histological findings of the skin injuries are presented below.

For the finding of metallization, both extensive deposits of foreign material on the intact epidermis and deposits in the skin with destruction of the epidermis and tuft-like elongation of basal cells were found, as were also observed in electrical marks caused by technical electricity (Pollak et al. 1988). In another lightning accident with tattoo-like deposition of gold, silver, and copper in the victim's skin, the necklace worn at the time of the lightning strike had completely evaporated. Six months after the event, a skin biopsy showed histiocytes, fibroblasts, and multinucleated foreign body giant cells in the immediate vicinity of the foreign particles, both in the skin and in the subcutaneous fat tissue (Jonas et al. 2002). In a similar accident caused by lightning strike, granulomas with foreign body giant cells were also described (Saleem et al. 2013).

A histologically examined lightning exit mark on a victim's foot showed destruction of the dermis with central necrosis and peripheral vacuolation (Pollak et al. 1988).

In an examination of a Lichtenberg figure, dilations of the blood and lymph vessels as well as intravascular platelet aggregation were found (Pollak et al. 1988).

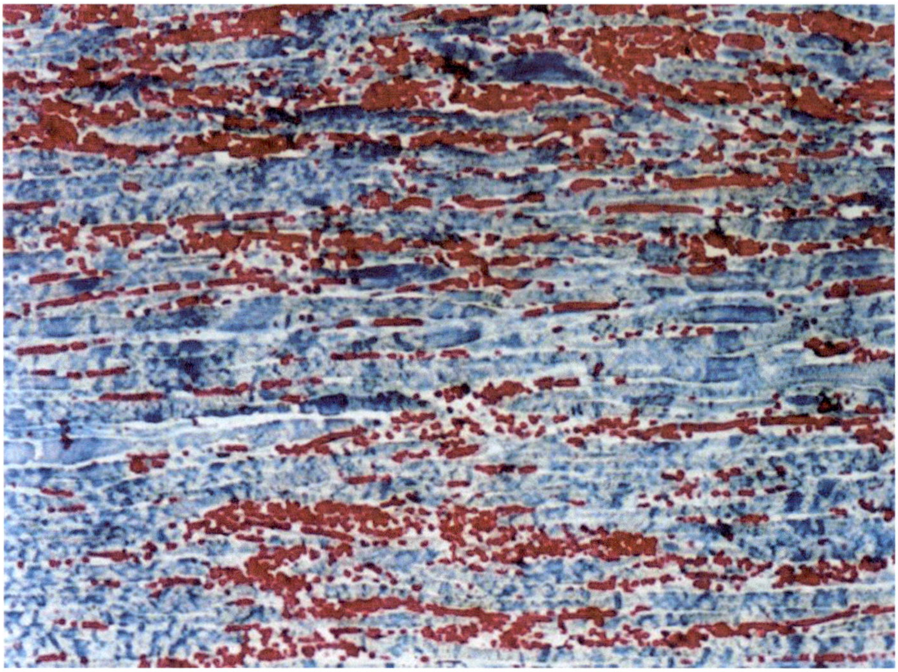

Fig. 7.28 Preferentially stripe-shaped hemorrhages in the interstitium of the myocardium 5 days after a lightning strike (CAB, 56:1). (Own illustration)

The microscopic analysis of a lightning-induced burn of the skin showed a blister-like lifting of the epidermis from the dermis without cellular reaction (Wetli 1996).

Even though the diagnosis of death by lightning strike is often made by a careful external post-mortem examination, performed autopsies can lead to a better understanding of the pathophysiology of death and in overlooked cases also to the correct diagnosis (Cherington et al. 2001; Zack et al. 1997). Against this background, the negative development of autopsy rates in Germany that has been observed for many years is alarming. It is therefore not surprising that in the last 20 years, with one exception, no autopsies had taken place in all other fatal lightning accidents from Germany published in medical journals (Möhle et al. 2015; Püschel et al. 2009; Zack et al. 2010, 2013).

Possibilities and Limitations of Autopsy in Death by Lightning Strike

- There are lightning accidents that could only be clarified by an autopsy.
- There are no morphological findings that occur in every case of a lightning strike with health damage to a person.

- The possible forms of energy transferred in a lightning accident can lead to a wide variety of possible pathomorphological findings.
- After a survived or initially survived lightning accident, acute myocardial necroses are often observed. In these cases, the victims usually show no pathological findings on the coronary arteries.
- There is no histological finding that is pathognomonic for the diagnosis *death by lightning strike* on its own.

7.4 Epidemiological Data

In the professional literature there are various epidemiological data about injuries caused by lightning strikes in different countries of the world. The actual number of worldwide annual deaths and injuries is, as expected, not known. The documented number of people

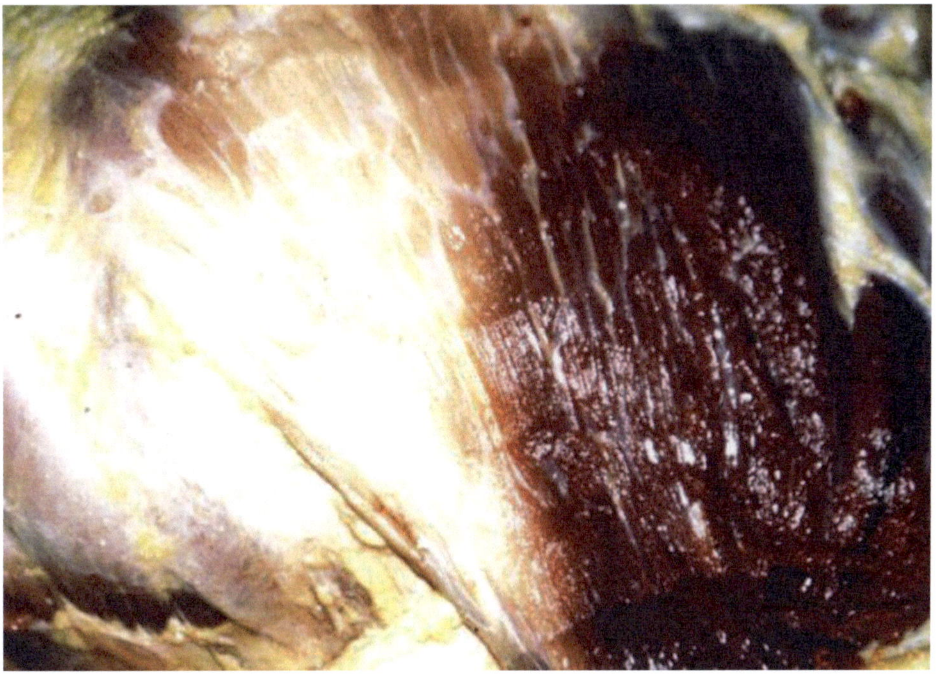

Fig. 7.29 Coagulation of parts of the left pectoralis major muscle under intact skin 5 days after an accident by side flash. (Own illustration)

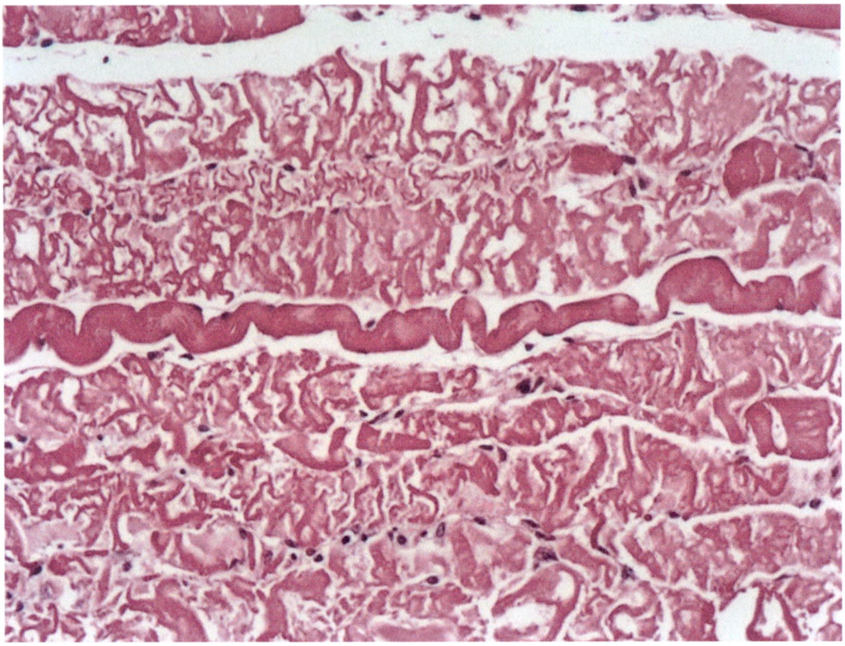

Fig. 7.30 Areactive necrosis of the left pectoralis major muscle, same case as Fig. 7.29 (HE, 112:1). (Own illustration)

who have died from lightning strikes worldwide is currently estimated at over 4000–6000 cases per year based on published national datasets. Taking into account numerous missing data, especially from developing countries, which are often located in a region with a high frequency of thunderstorms, a frequency of up to 24,000 fatal accidents caused by lightning strikes per year is to be expected (Blumenthal 2018; Cooper and Holle 2019; Guha et al. 2021).

In human medicine, incidence is often defined as the number of new cases occurring in a population and a year per 100,000 people. In contrast, when evaluating fatal lightning accidents in international comparison, it has proven useful to calculate the incidence of people killed in a year and country per 1 million inhabitants.

7.4.1 Frequency and Incidence

Germany

Using the cause of death statistics from the Federal Statistical Office, Schniers (2005) evaluated the deaths caused by lightning strikes from 1950–1989 for the Federal Republic of Germany. A steady decline in fatal accidents was observed. While between 33 and 101 deaths of this type of accident were registered annually in the period from 1950–1959, the number of people killed by lightning strikes in the period from 1980–1989 dropped to 2–19 per year. Since there was also an increase in the population in the Federal Republic of Germany in the period from 1950–1989, the incidence of the deceased per 1 million inhabitants in this period decreased from 1.71 for 1950 to 0.03 for 1989 (Table 7.5). Since then, the number of people killed by lightning has settled at a low level, usually below 10 cases per year (proportions of the world population 2023; Federal Statistical Office Germany 2020; Zack et al. 2009).

Other Developed Countries

This positive development in terms of the incidence of lethal lightning accidents is similar in other developed countries. For example, the incidence of this cause of death in the USA fell from 6.6 for the year 1900 to 0.1 for 2010. In absolute numbers, this means for the United States of America that the number of deaths caused by lightning has reduced from over 400 fatalities per year around 1900 to under 30 annually after 2000, despite an increase in population (Adekoya and Nolte 2005; Holle 2015). Similar developments have occurred in other European countries and Canada (Table 7.6) (Cooper and Holle 2019).

Causes for the Decline in Fatal Lightning Accidents in Developed Countries

This continuous decline in deaths from lightning injuries in developed countries obviously has multifactorial causes.

One reason is the increase in buildings as relatively safe places, which nowadays usually have at least an internal lightning protection system. This system consists of metallic installations, electrical and electronic systems, lightning protection potential equalization and separation distance, and is designed to prevent a dangerous spark formation within the facility to be protected. The external lightning protection system, which is based on an invention by the American scientist and politician Benjamin Franklin and is visible from the outside, consists of a lightning rod, a down conductor, and a grounding electrode (Heidler and Stimper 2009; Uman 1986, 2008).

Table 7.5 Deaths by lightning strike per 1 million inhabitants in the Federal Republic of Germany from 1950–1989. (Own representation)

Year	Deaths by lightning strike	Population (Million)	Deaths per 1 Million inhabitants
1950	86	50.336	1.71
1960	29	55.787	0.52
1970	25	61.001	0.41
1980	11	61.658	0.18
1989	2	62.679	0.03

Table 7.6 Incidences of lethal lightning accidents per 1 million inhabitants, period and region as indicated in the specialist literature. (Own representation)

Country/City-State/Region	Year/Period	Incidence	Authors
USA	1900	6.6	Cooper and Holle 2019
South Africa	1997–2000	6.3	Blumenthal 2005
Mexico	1979–2011	2.7	Raga et al. 2014
Wyoming	1968–1985	1.96	Duclos and Sanderson 1990
Colombia	2000–2009	1.78	Navarrete and Rodriguez 2016
Germany	1950	1.71	Bremer 2024
Singapore	1961–1979	1.7	Pakiam et al. 1981
England and Wales	1852–1859	1.13	Elsom 2001
Bangladesh	2003	0.9	Biswas et al. 2016
USA	1959–1994	0.42	Curran et al. 2000
England and Wales	1900–1909	0.41	Elsom 2001
USA	1995–2002	0.23	Adekoya and Nolte 2005
Sweden	1975–1984	0.2	Eriksson and Örnehult 1988
Canada	1990–2004	0.2	Mills et al. 2006
USA	2010	0.1	Cooper et al. 2017
England and Wales	1990–1999	0.05	Elsom 2001
Germany	1999	0.01	Krause 2004
Australia	1980–1989	0.001	Coates et al. 1993

Another reason is the increasing registration rates of motor vehicles with metal roofs over the past decades, which act as a Faraday cage in the event of a lightning strike and protect the occupants from injuries caused by the electric current.

Considering the large number of fatal accidents caused by lightning strikes during various unprotected activities in agriculture in the last century, the introduction of machines with driver's cabins and the simultaneous reduction in the number of employees in the past decades have been significant factors in the decline of those killed by lightning in developed nations.

Other causes are likely to be improved first aid and emergency medical care at the accident site, faster transport of a severely injured victim to a suitable clinic, and better treatment options through modern intensive care medicine.

But also the expansion of specialist knowledge and the role of modern media in disseminating knowledge about the correct behavior during a thunderstorm should not be overlooked as contributing reasons. Last but not least, professional weather forecasts and the technical possibilities of potentially receiving information about short-term weather changes and storm warnings should be mentioned in this context.

Developing Countries

While the reported incidences of fatal lightning accidents in developed countries and in recent decades have always been below 1, this positive development does not apply worldwide. For example, Cooper and Holle (2019) report incidences of 14–84 for the developing countries Zimbabwe and Malawi after 1979, without however specifying the exact recording period. But also the incidences for South Africa (6.3 for 1997–2000), Mexico (2.7 for 1979–2011) and Colombia (1.78 for 2000–2009) are far above the reported numbers for the countries of Europe and North America in the comparable period (Table 7.6).

If one considers the previously mentioned, most likely causal factors for the decline in fatal lightning accidents in developed countries, it becomes obvious that these favored reasons cannot be transferred to developing countries. For countries with high incidence rates of deaths from lightning strikes, it is additionally problematic that they often lie in the tropical climate zone and thus have a much higher lightning density per square kilometer and unit of time than developed countries, which are predominantly located in the temperate climate zone (Cooper et al. 2017). Therefore, it is not only welcome from a medical point of view that international interdisciplinary lightning research has increasingly taken on the task of lightning protection and educating the population in developing countries in recent years (Cooper et al. 2017; Cooper and Holle 2019; Gomes and Gomes 2021; Guha et al. 2021; Holle et al. 2021).

7.4.2 Gender Distribution

That of the 237 victims of lightning strikes in Germany in the period from 1980–2000, with 82.2% of the cases, the male gender was significantly more affected than the female, is no surprise (Schniers 2005). In an evaluation of published studies with specific information about case numbers and study periods from various nations, proportions

Table 7.7 Proportion of male victims in fatal accidents due to lightning strikes. (Own illustration)

Total number of victims	Number of male victims	Relative frequency (in %)	Country/Region	Time period	Authors
44	40	90.9	USA	1958–1994	Wetli 1996
101	88	87.1	Florida	1978–1987	Duclos et al. 1990
1916	1629	85	USA	1968–1985	Duclos and Sanderson 1990
236	194	82.2	Germany	1980–2000	Schniers 2005
757	608	80.3	Colombia	2000–2009	Navarrete-Aldana et al. 2014
38	30	78.8	South Africa	1997–2000	Blumenthal 2005
19	15	78.9	Sweden	1975–1984	Eriksson and Örnehult 1988
22	16	72.7	United Kingdom	1993–1999	Elsom 2001

of the male gender of 72.7–90.9% were found (Table 7.7). One reason for the significant difference in gender distribution may be that men work outdoors more often than women. Another reason could be an increased risk-taking behavior of male individuals compared to females (Diehl 2008).

Case Study

On a June day in 2008, 17 men and 3 women were undergoing football coaching training under a 44-year-old teacher on a football field in North Rhine-Westphalia (Germany). As thunderclouds gathered in the late morning, 16 men were still on the field training. The football teacher considered whether he should call it off. He decided against an early termination of the exercises and continued training. The teacher and several other men saw a bluish flash before the lightning struck the ground of the sports field, injuring numerous men through the step voltage they had received. The spectrum of health damage ranged from immediate unconsciousness to persistent pain, without further details being provided. After the arrival of the rescue teams, 5 male participants were admitted to a clinic, all of whom survived the lightning strike accident. The 3 participating women had moved to relatively safe places in time and remained unharmed (Diehl 2008; Zack et al. 2009). ◀

▶ **Note** In lethal lightning accidents, the male gender is significantly more often affected.

7.4.3 Distribution by Age

A study on the age of victims of lethal lightning accidents in Germany for the period from 1980–2000 showed that children under 10 years and older people over 70 years died relatively rarely from this type of accident. The decade from 10 to under 20 years had the most victims with 59 (24.9%) fatalities, followed by the age groups 20 to under 30 years with 42 (17.7%) and 30 to under 40 years with 37 (15.6%) fatalities (Schniers 2005).

Compared to information on the gender distribution of killed lightning victims, there were fewer reports on age distributions in the specialist literature. Moreover, the age categories often differ from study to study, so direct comparisons, such as in the case of gender distribution, are not readily possible. Nevertheless, it is noticeable in almost all published studies that younger people are most often affected by lethal lightning accidents. Thus, Mills et al. (2006) state that 51% of all killed lightning victims in Canada in the period from 1986–2005 were aged 16–45 years. In Singapore, 58% of the fatalities from 1922–1979 were aged 10–29 years (Pakiam et al. 1981). Without naming specific numbers, Coates et al. (1993) found a concentration among 15- to 34-year-olds for Australia, Thacker et al. (2008) among 20- to 34-year-olds for the USA, and Navarrete-Aldana et al. (2014) among 11- to 45-year-old victims for Colombia. However, these studies only considered the total number of deceased persons. A consideration of the percentage of the formed age groups in the total population was first made in 2017 in an epidemiological study from Bangladesh. While the absolute numbers showed the 20–29 age group to be most frequently affected, a consideration of the percentage shares of the formed age groups in the total population of the country showed that the 30–39 age group had the most deaths from lightning strikes (Dewan et al. 2017).

The reasons why younger people in developed countries are more often affected by a lethal lightning strike than older people are obviously also due to the leisure behavior of the different age groups. When playing, doing sports, and other leisure activities outdoors, people of the younger age groups are likely to be found more often and thus be potential victims than the older generation. On the other hand, knowledge about proper behavior in case of thunderstorm danger and risk-taking also play a role in the mentioned results regarding age distribution.

However, younger people are also more often affected than older ones in developing countries. Here, the statistics are burdened, among other things, by numerous accidents in schools, especially in African countries, as the school buildings are often open and have neither an internal nor an external lightning protection system (Cooper and Holle 2019).

> **Note** Younger people are more often involved in lethal accidents caused by lightning strikes than older ones.

7.4.4 Temporal Distribution

Daily Distribution

There is a maximum of lethal accidentsby lightning strike in the afternoon and evening hours, and a minimum in the night and morning hours of a day. These results of numerous studies apply to both the northern and southern hemispheres of the earth. Both Duclos and Sanderson (1990) for the USA (study scope: 1916 cases) and Blumenthal (2005) for South Africa (38 cases) consistently report a clustering of such deaths between 3:00 pm and 8:00 pm local time. However, there are also results that deviate slightly from this. For example, Wetli (1996) describes a peak at 2 pm for the US state of Florida (45 cases). The mentioned daily accumulations of deaths by lightning strike in the USA correspond with the daily distribution of the frequency of cloud-to-ground lightning for the territory of the country, even though this statistic was only collected for the period 2005–2012. Holle (2014) reports in his evaluation of the data of the National Lightning Detection Network of the USA a clustering of these lightning strikes from 12:00 pm to 12:00 am.

Distribution by Days of the Week

Compared to the daily and monthly distribution, there are only a few studies in the literature about the distribution of lethal lightning accidents by days of the week. In a study of 53 deaths in Canada, the most fatal lightning strikes were found on a Saturday with n = 14 (26.4%) (Mills et al. 2006). A study from Sweden with an even smaller number of cases showed that of 18 lethal lightning accidents, 4 (22.2%) occurred on a Saturday or Sunday (Eriksson and Örnehult 1988). These results could be a discreet indication that leisure activities on weekends in appropriate weather conditions pose an increased risk for lethal lightning accidents.

Monthly Distribution

In all countries with epidemiological data on lethal accidents caused by lightning strikes, there is a clustering of such events in the warm season, when the number of heat thunderstorms is naturally highest (see chap. 3). For example, in Germany and large parts of Europe and North America, which are located in the temperate climate zone, these are particularly the months of May to September and in numerous nations of the southern hemisphere of the earth the months of November to March (Blumenthal 2005; Coates et al. 1993; Duclos and Sanderson 1990; Mills et al. 2006; Schniers 2005; Wetli 1996). For countries with tropical or subtropical climates, this assessment does not apply. For example, in a study of 757 deaths in Colombia from 2000–2009, lethal accidents were found in all 12 months, with a significant reduction in fatal events only in the months of January and February. On the other hand, the most deaths were found in the months of April and October (Navarrete-Aldana et al. 2014).

> **Note** In Germany and other countries of the temperate climate zone in the northern hemisphere of the earth, lethal lightning accidents occur most frequently in the afternoon or evening hours of the day in the months of May to September.

7.4.5 Activities of the Victims and Accident Locations

Activities

There is a study in the German-speaking specialist literature by Harms (1956), which provides concrete numbers about the activities and the locations of the victims of a lightning strike at the time of the accident. The engineer from Hanover evaluated an inhomogeneous collection of information about lightning accidents, organized by the Committee for Lightning Rod Construction in the United Economic Area e. V., which had occurred in Germany in the period from 1950–1955. In this, he found information about the activities of the victims at the time of the accident for 135 out of 173 fatalities. The accumulation of lethal accidents due to lightning strikes in agriculture, where many people used to work unprotected outdoors, was also shown in the results of studies by other scientists (Cooper and Holle 2019; Holle et al. 2005). However, there are numerous other activities at the times of the accidents, which are often divided into indoor and outdoor activities. For example, activities outside of buildings include horse riding, camping, mountaineering, fishing, and visiting the circus. Activities inside buildings include using a corded telephone, sleeping, or standing at an open window or door (Andrews 1992; Blanco-Pampin et al. 1997; Dinakaran et al. 1998; Holle et al. 2005; Mills et al. 2006). In the aforementioned older study from Germany, 7 fatalities were reported during sports activities without listing the individual sports (Harms 1956). In contrast, the sports of golf, football, baseball, and horse riding are particularly mentioned in the specialist literature. There have been numerous severe lightning accidents worldwide among golfers and footballers while practicing their sports (Cherington et al. 1998; Dollinger 1985; Mills et al. 2006; Zack et al. 2009, 2013).

Accident Locations

The places where people in developed countries have most frequently died from lightning strikes have changed over time. More than 100 years ago, victims of such accidents preferred to die on a field, pasture, or in a building. Statistical surveys in recent decades from the USA have shown that there are hardly any deaths in enclosed buildings nowadays and a significant decrease in lethal accidents due to lightning strikes in connection with unprotected work in agriculture. On the other hand, deaths outdoors, especially during sports and recreation, have increased (Holle et al. 2005; Walsh et al. 2013). Thus, there has been a panorama change regarding the locations of fatal lightning strike accidents (Cooper and Holle 2019). In the already cited study from Germany for the period from 1950–1955, 24.8% of the accidents were found under free-standing trees and also 24.8% while staying in an open area. On streets and paths (14.9%), there were also relatively frequent deaths from lightning strikes at that time, as well as in unfinished new buildings (8.1%) (Harms 1956). Bremer (2024) states in her dissertation that 32.2% of the evaluated 270 lethal lightning accidents in Germany between 1951–1965 occurred under free-standing trees. The fatal accidents occurred under 19 different types of trees, most frequently under spruces (15 cases), poplars (12 cases), and oaks (10 cases). The 5 lethal events that were demonstrably found under beech trees make the in Germany widely spread saying "You should seek beeches, but avoid oaks" absurd.

With the introduction of modern lightning protection systems in house construction and the industrialization of agriculture, there has been both a significant decrease in the incidences of death by lightning strike and a change in the potentially most dangerous places in developed countries (Cooper and Holle 2019). In none of the mentioned studies have deaths by lightning strike under bridges been reported so far (see chap. 8).

7.4.6 Case Numbers per Lightning Accident

In an accident caused by a lightning strike, there can be just one, a few, or many victims. A significant difference is observed in the number of people killed or injured by lightning per event between developed and developing countries, as well as in the different activities of people. For example, in the USA from 1959–1994, 91% of lightning accidents resulted in only one person being killed and 68% resulted in only one person being injured (Curran et al. 2000). In England and Wales, 98% and in Singapore 72% of accidents with only one person killed were reported (Elsom and Webb 2014; Pakiam et al. 1981). However, if we only consider accidents during leisure activities or sports, the relative proportion of accidents with only one person killed drops to 31% (Cooper and Holle 2019).

In developing countries, there are much more frequent accidents caused by lightning with multiple fatalities and/or injuries. Schools and agricultural fields are the preferred locations for accidents with numerous victims. For agriculturally used locations, a relative proportion of accidents with only one fatality of only 50% is reported, while this proportion drops to 39% for lethal events in schools (Cooper and Holle 2019).

7.5 Lethality

The term lethality describes the fatal disease courses in relation to the total frequency of a defined disease (Pschyrembel 2020). Taking into account a previously defined period, lethality is also defined as the ratio of the number of deaths from a particular disease to the total number of new cases (Kundt et al. 2012). Since there is no comparable category for accidents in human medicine, the term lethality is also applied to these events, such as death by lightning strike (Puchstein 2016; Zack et al. 2016).

A correct calculation of lethality after personal injuries caused by lightning is not possible for various reasons. On the one hand, there are deaths caused by lightning that are overlooked by the medical examiner and therefore do not enter the corresponding statistics. On the other hand, there are no reliable figures for surviving victims. While there is no official statistic for survivors of lightning accidents in Germany, figures on the number of surviving accident victims have been published in the USA and Great Britain. However, the publications show that the figures are composed from various sources and are by no means complete (Cooray et al. 2007; Elsom and Webb 2014).

> ▶ **Note** The lethality of lightning accidents has decreased in recent decades and is currently between 8 and 27%.

The information on the lethality of accidents caused by lightning varies greatly in the technical literature and ranges from 3–90% (Gurr and Brown 1998; Hinkelbein et al. 2013; Keil 2009; Kupfer et al. 1987; Muehlberger et al. 2001; Zimmermann et al. 2002). In German forensic textbooks, 30–40% is often stated (Dettmeyer and Verhoff 2011; Penning 2006; Pollak 2007; Reimann and Prokop 1980; Schwerd 1992; Sellier 1975). In Anglo-American literature, reports of 20–30% are preferred (Carleton 1995; Cooper 1995; Cooper et al. 2001; Hauser et al. 2013; Lifschultz and Donoghue 1993a; Sanford and Gamelli 2014). In Japan, however, a lethality of 80% was mentioned (Hayashi et al.

2005). Sources for these figures were generally not found. This high discrepancy in the literature led to a scientific review at the Rostock Institute for Forensic Medicine (Germany), the results of which were published in 2016 (Puchstein 2016; Zack et al.2016). In this process, scientific publications were evaluated using a selective literature search, which provided specific statistical data for victims of a lightning strike accident in a defined period for a country or a large city. On the other hand, scientific papers were analyzed that reported on lightning accidents with more than one victim. All events involving harm to only one person were excluded in the Rostock study because publications in medical journals are made according to certain criteria, such as the rarity of findings or new results, and thus an unwanted selection of cases had been made in advance. The evaluation of the published statistics yielded a total of 19,444 people who had been harmed by a lightning strike. Of these, 5,103 victims died, so the lethality of this group was 26.2% (Table 7.8). The analysis of the 102 lightning accidents with more than one victim published in professional journals resulted in a total of 1,256 injured people, of whom 105 died. The calculated lethality of this study group was 8.4% (Puchstein 2016).

Table 7.8 Information on lethality in lightning strike accidents based on statistical surveys. (Own representation)

Period	Country/City/Region	Total accident victims	Deceased accident victims	Lethality in %	Authors
1975–1998	Ankara	22	0	0	Aslar et al. 2001
2005–2015	Austria/Alps	64	4	6.2	Ströhle et al. 2018
1988–2012	United Kingdom	722	47	6.5	Elsom and Webb 2014
1965–1999	Japan	312	56	17.9	Ohashi et al. 2001
1949–1959	Budapest	26	5	19.2	Iranyi et al. 1962
n. s	n. s	221	43	19.5	Andrews et al. 1989
2007–2011	Uganda	734	150	20.4	Mary and Gomes 2012
1959–1994	USA	13,057	3239	24.8	Curran et al. 2000
1965–1969	Austria	162	48	29.6	Karobath et al. 1971
n. s	n. s	66	20	30.3	Cooper 1980
1959–1960	Hungary	156	50	32.0	Iranyi et al. 1962
1950–1958	USA	2373	828	34.9	Uman 1986
1965–1999	Japan	1125	440	39.1	Ohashi et al. 2001
1950–1955	FRG	404	173	42.8	Harms 1956
Total		**19,444**	**5,103**	**26.2**	

n. s. not specified

On the Lethality of Accidents Caused by Lightning Strikes

- The assessment of the probability that a person will die after a lightning strike accident is of considerable relevance for accident prevention, insurance law issues, and professional knowledge.
- A lethality of 80–90% for all accidents caused by lightning strikes with personal injuries is not comprehensible after scientific review of the data.
- The lethality for lightning strike accidents of 30–90% stated in German-speaking forensic medical textbooks is no longer correct. After an analysis of the professional literature of the last decades, a lethality between 8% and 27% is to be assumed.
- Publications with a stated lethality of over 30% date back several decades. In more recent publications, a lower lethality is found. This trend is most likely due to improved first aid and emergency medical care for the victims.

References

Adekoya N, Nolte KB (2005) Struck-by-lightning deaths in the United States. J Environ Health 67:45–50

Alyan O, Ozdemir O, Tufekcioglu O, Geyik B, Aras D, Demirkan D (2006) Myocardial injury due to lightning strike—a case report. Angiology 57:219–223

Amy BW, McManus WF, Goodwin CW, Pruitt BA (1985) Lightning injury with survival in five patients. JAMA 253:243–245

Andrews CJ (1992) Telephone related lightning injury. Med J Australia 157:823–826

Andrews CJ, Cooper MA (1992) Clinical presentations of the lightning victim. In: Andrews CJ, Cooper MA, Darvenzia M, Mackerras D (eds) Lightning injuries: electrical, medical, and legal aspects. CRC Press, Boca Raton, pp 47–70

Andrews CJ, Reisner AD (2017) Neurological and neurophysiological consequences of electrical and lightning shock: review and theories of causation. Neural Regen Res 12:677–686

Andrews CJ, Darveniza M, Mackerras D (1989) Lightning injury: a review of clinical aspects, pathophysiology and treatment. Adv Trauma 4:241–252

Apanga PA, Azumah JA, Yiranbon JB (2017) A rare manifestation of burns after lightning strike in rural Ghana: a case report. J Med Case Rep 11:200

Arden GP, Harrison SH, Lister J, Maudsley RH (1956) Lightning accident at Ascot. BMJ 4981:1450–1453

Arnould JF, Le Floch R (2011) Lichtenberg figures associated with a high-voltage industrial burn. Burns 37:e13–e15

Aslar AK, Soran A, Yildiz Y, Isik Y (2001) Epidemiology, morbidity, mortality and treatment of lightning injuries in a Turkish burns units. Int J Clin Pract 55:502–504

Aydin F, Yildrim OT, Dagtekin E, Aydin AH, Aksit E (2018) Acute inferior myocardial infarction caused by lightning strike. Prehosp Disaster Med 33:658–659

Badagliacca P, Gentile L, Marruchella G (2017) Pathology in practice. J Am Vet Med Assoc 250:859–861

Bartholome CW, Jacoby WD, Ramchand SC (1975) Cutaneous manifestations of lightning injury. Arch Dermatol 111:1466–1468

Bartsch A (2013) Strom- und Blitzunfall. Notfall Rettungsmed 16:643–652

Bingert R, Bremer L, Büttner A, Nigbur S, Blumenthal R, Zack F (2024) A 15-year review of lightning deaths in Germany—with a focus on pathognomonic findings. Int J Legal Med 138: 1343–1349

Biswas A, Dalal K, Hossain J, Baset KU, Rahman F, Mashreky SR (2016) Lightning injury is a disaster in Bangladesh?—Exploring its magnitude and public health needs (version 1; referees: 3 approved, 1 approved with reservations). F1000Research 5:2931

Blanco-Pampin JM, Suarez-Penaranda JM, Rico-Boquete R, Concheira-Carro L (1997) An unusual case of death by lightning. J Forensic Sci 42:942–944

Blumenthal R (2005) Lightning fatalities on the South African Highveld: a retrospective descriptive study for the period 1997 to 2000. Am J Forensic Med Pathol 26:66–69

Blumenthal R (2012) Secondary missile injury from lightning strike. Am J Forensic Med Pathol 33:83–85

Blumenthal R (2018) Lightning and the forensic pathologist. Acad Forensic Pathol 8:98–111

Blumenthal R (2021) Injuries and deaths from lightning. J Clin Pathol 74:279–284

Blumenthal R (2022) Electrocution and lightning. In: Madea B (ed) Handbook of forensic medicine. vol 2, 2nd edn. Wiley, Chichester

Blumenthal R, Saayman G (2017) Case report: lightning-induced pneumomediastinum. Am J Forensic Med Pathol 38:94–96

Bremer L (2024) Retrospektive Analyse einer historischen Fallsammlung von letalen Unfällen durch Blitzschlag in der Bundesrepublik Deutschland im Zeitraum 1951–1965 aus rechtsmedizinischer Sicht. Med Diss. Universität Rostock, Rostock

Browne BJ, Gaasch WR (1992) Electrical injuries and lightning. Emerg Med Clin North Am 10:211–229

Byard RW (2023) Lichtenberg figures—morphological findings. Forensic Sci Med Pathol 19:269–272

Carleton SC (1995) Cardiac problems associated with electrical injury. Cardiol Clin 13:263–266

Carte AE, Anderson RB, Cooper MA (2002) A large group of children struck by lightning. Ann Emerg Med 39:665–670

Chao TC (1984) Lightning deaths in Singapore. Acta Med Leg Soc Liege 34:129–131

Cherington M, Yarnell PR, Todd HM (1994) Lightning injury and glioma. Int J Care Inj 25:687–688

Cherington M, Yarnell PR, London SF (1995) Neurologic complications of lightning injuries. West J Med 162:413–417

Cherington M, Krider EP, Yarnell PR, Breed DW (1997) A bolt from the blue: lightning strike to the head. Neurology 48:683–686

Cherington M, Wachtel H, Yarnell PR (1998) Could lightning injury be magnetically induced? Lancet 351:1788

Cherington M, Kurtzman R, Krider EP, Yarnell PR (2001) Mountain medical mystery. Unwitnessed death of a healthy young man, caused by lightning. Am J Forensic Med Pathol 22:296–298

Cherington M, Olson S, Yarnell PR (2003) Lightning and Lichtenberg figures. Injury 34:367–371

Coates L, Blong R, Siciliano F (1993) Lightning fatalities in Australia, 1824–1991. Nat Hazards 8:217–233

Cooper MA (1980) Lightning injuries: prognostic signs for death. Ann Emerg Med 9:134–138

Cooper MA (1995) Myths, miracles, and mirages. Semin Neurol 15:358–361

Cooper MA, Holle RL (2019) Reducing lightning injuries worldwide. Springer, Cham

Cooper MA, Andrews CJ, Holle RL, Lopez R (2001) Lightning injuries. In: Auerbach PS (ed) Wilderness medicine: management of wilderness and environmental emergencies. 4th edn. Mosby, St. Louis, pp 74–76

Cooper MA, Andrews CJ, Holle RL, Blumenthal R, Navarette-Aldana N (2017) Lightning-related injuries and safety. In: Auerbach P, Cushing T, Harris N (eds) Auerbach's wilderness medicine. 7th edn. Elsevier, Philadelphia, pp 71–117

Cooray V, Cooray C, Andrews CJ (2007) Lightning caused injuries in humans. J Electrostatics 65:386–394

Courtman SP, Wilson PM, Mok Q (2003) Case report of a 13-year-old struck by lightning. Paediatr Anaesth 13:76–79

Curran EB, Holle RL, Lopez RE (2000) Lightning casualities and damages in the United States from 1959 to 1994. J Climate 13:3448–3464

Davidson GS, Deck JH (1988) Delayed myelopathy following lightning strike: a demyelinating process. Acta Neuropathol 77:104–108

Dettmeyer RB (2018) Forensic Histopathology. Fundamentals and Perspectives. Springer, Heidelberg

Dettmeyer RB, Verhoff MA (2011) Rechtsmedizin. Springer, Heidelberg

Dewan A, Hossain F, Rahman M, Yamane Y, Holle RL (2017) Recent lightning-related fatalities and injuries in Bangladesh. Weather Clim Soc 9:575–589

Diehl J (2008) Eine Meldung und ihre Geschichte—warum ein Blitz 19 Fußballtrainer gleichzeitig traf. Spiegel 27:55

Diepenseifen CJ, Schewe JC, Malotki F, Conrad H (2009) Blitzunfall bei Flugschau. Notfall Rettungsmed 12:523–530

Dinakaran S, Desai SP, Elsom DM (1998) Telephon-mediated lightning injury causing cataract. Injury 29:645–646

Dollinger SJ (1985) Lightning-strike disaster among children. Br J Med Psychol 58:375–383

Domart N (2000) Lichtenberg figures due to lightning strike. N Engl J Med 343:1536

Duclos PJ, Sanderson LM (1990) An epidemiological description of lightning-related deaths in the United States. Int J Epidemiol 19:673–679

Duclos PJ, Sanderson LM, Klontz KC (1990) Lightning-related mortality and morbidity in Florida. Public Health Rep 105:276–282

ten Duis HJ (1992) Musculoskeletal system and skin, including burns. In: Andrews CJ, Cooper MA, Darvenzia M, Mackerras D (eds) Lightning injuries: electrical, medical, and legal aspects. CRC Press, Boca Raton, pp 101–111

ten Duis HJ, Klasen HJ, Nijsten MWN, Pietronero L (1987) Superficial lightning injuries: their "fractal" shape and origin. Burns 13:141–146

Duppel H, Löbermann M, Reisinger EC (2009) Aus heiterem Himmel vom Blitz getroffen. Dtsch Med Wochenschr 134:1214–1217

Dürwald W (1986) Gerichtliche Medizin 2nd edn. Barth, Leipzig

Dutta B (2016) Lichtenberg figure and lightning. Indian J Dermatol 61:109–111

Eadie MJ (1992) Pathophysiology of lightning injury to the nervous system. In: Andrews CJ, Cooper MA, Darvenzia M, Mackerras D (eds) Lightning injuries: electrical, medical, and legal aspects. CRC Press, Boca Raton, pp 81–86

Ebertz M (1891) Ueber Blitzschlagverletzungen. Dtsch Med Wochenschr 36:1848–1852

Ekoe JM, Cunnigham M, Jaques O, Balgue F, Baumann RP, Humair L, de Torrente A (1985) Disseminated intravascular coagulation and acute myocardial necrosis caused by lightning. Intensive Care Med 11:160–162

Elsom DM (2001) Deaths and injuries caused by lightning in the United Kingdom: analyses of two databases. Atmos Res 56:325–334

Elsom DM, Webb JDC (2014) Death and injuries from lightning in the UK, 1988–2012. Weather 69:221–226

Eriksson A, Örnehult L (1988) Death by lightning. Am J Forensic Med Pathol 9:295–300

Figgis P, Alvarez G (2012) Delayed esophageal perforation following lightning strike: a case report and review of the literature. J Med Case Rep 6:244

Forster SA, Silva IM, Ramos MLC, Gragnani A, Ferreira LM (2013) Lightning burn—review and case report. Burns 39:e8–e12

Geary SP, Spencer T, Tilney PVR (2015) A 26-year-old man struck by lightning. Air Med J 34:8–11

Gomes C, Gomes A (2021) Public concepts and safety education. In: Gomes C (ed) Lightning. Science, engineering, and economic implications for developing countries. Springer, Singapore, pp 275–300

Gruhn KM, Knossalla F, Schwenkreis P, Hamsen U, Schildhauer TA, Tegenthoff M, Sczesny-Kaiser M (2016) Neurologische Erkrankungen nach Blitzschlag. Lightning strikes twice. Nervenarzt 87:623–628

Guha A, Liu Y, Williams E, Schumann C, Hunt H (2021) Lightning detection and warning. In: Gomes C (ed) Lightning. Science, engineering, and economic implications for developing countries. Springer, Singapore, pp 37–77

Gurr DE, Brown TC (1998) Zapped—recognition and treatment of lightning strike and electrical injuries. JEMS 23:66–74

Hanson GC, McIlwraith GR (1973) Lightning injury: two case histories and a review of management. Br Med J 4:271–274

Harms W (1956) Personenblitzschäden. Elektromedizin 1:153–158

Harms W (1961) Personenblitzschäden 1959 in der Bundesrepublik. Elektromedizin 6:44

Harwood SJ, Catrou PG, Cole W (1978) Creatine phosphokinase isoenzyme fractions in the serum of a patient struck by lightning. Arch Intern Med 138:645–646

Hauser R, Kaliszan M, Basir A, Basir ID (2013) Lightning strike as probable cause of death and determining identity based on the examination of skeletal remains. J Forensic Sci 58:527–529

Hayashi M, Yamada H, Aqatsuma T, Nomura H, Kitahara O (2005) A case of takotsubo-shaped hypokinesis of the left ventricle caused by a lightning strike. Int Heart J 46:933–938

Heidler F, Stimper K (2009) Blitz und Blitzschutz. VDE, Berlin Offenbach

Herold K (1960) Der Elektrotod. In: Prokop O (ed) Lehrbuch der gerichtlichen Medizin. Volk und Wissen, Berlin, pp 127–141

Hinkelbein J, Spelten O, Wetsch WA (2013) Blitzschlag und Blitzunfälle in der präklinischen Notfallmedizin. Unfallchirurg 116:74–79

Holle RL (2010) Lightning-caused casualities in and near dwellings and other buildings. https://www.vaisala.com/sites/default/files/documents/9.Holle-Lightning-Caused.pdf. Accessed: 14 Dec 2022.

Holle RL (2014) Diurnal variations of NLDN-reported cloud-to-ground lightning in the United States. Mon Weather Rev 142:1037–1052

Holle RL (2015) Some aspects of global lightning impacts. https://www.weather.gov/media/safety/Global_Aspects_holle15.pdf. Accessed: 3 Jan 2023.

Holle RL, Lopez RE, Navarro BC (2005) Deaths, injuries, and damages from lightning in the United States in the 1890s in comparison with the 1990s. J Appl Meteorol 44:1563–1573

Holle RL, Cooper MA, Navarrete-Aldana N (2021) Lightning injury: occurrence and medical treatment. In: Gomes C (ed) Lightning. Science, engineering, and economic implications for developing countries. Springer, Singapore, pp 263–273

Hunt HGP, Blumenthal R, Nixon KJ, Gomes C (2020) A multidisciplinary forensic analysis of two lightning deaths observed in South Africa. Int J Disaster Risk Reduct 51:101814

Iranyi J, Orovecz B, Somogyi E, Iranyi K (1962) Das Blitztrauma in neuer Sicht. Münch Med Wochenschr 104:1496–1500

Janssen W (1984) Forensic Histopathology. Springer, Berlin

Jefferiss WRS (1876) Three cases of lightning-stroke. Br Med J 1:102

Jellinek S (1903) Elektropathologie: Die Erkrankungen durch Blitzschlag und elektrischen Strom in klinischer und forensischer Darstellung. Enke, Stuttgart

Jonas L, Fulda G, Nizze H, Zimmermann R, Gross G, Zack F, Kröning G, Holzhüter G, Haas HJ (2002) Detection of gold particles in the neck skin after lightning stroke with evaporation of an ornamental chain. Ultrastruct Pathol 26:153–159

Just T, Kramp B, Pau HW (2002) Blitzschlaginduzierte Verletzungen des Ohres. HNO 50:170–171

Kannan RY, Chester DL, Titley OG (2004) Combined Bennett's fracture subluxation and scapho-trapezio-trapezoidal dislocation secondary to lightning strike. J Trauma 57:1351–1353

Karadas S, Vuruskan E, Dursun R, Sincer I, Gonullu H, Akkaya E (2013) Myocardial infarction due to lightning strike. J Pak Med Assoc 63:1186–1188

Karobath H, Undt W, Hofschneider H (1971) Zur Wirkung des Blitzschlages auf den Organismus mit besonderer Berücksichtigung der Auswirkungen auf das Herz. Verh Dtsch Ges Inn Med 77:455–457

Karobath H, Redtenbacher M, Hofecker G, Walde I, Syre G (1977) Zur Frage der Todesursache beim Blitzunfall. Münch Med Wochenschr 119:29–32

Keil W (2009) Basics Rechtsmedizin, 1. Aufl. Elsevier Urban & Fischer, München

Kharoshah M, Alsaif DM, Albouijan A, Almoghannam S (2023) A rare case of fatal lightning strike in Dammam with unusual cutaneous findings. Saudi J Forensic Med Sci 3:32–35

Kilbas Z, Akin M, Gorgulu S, Mentes O, Ozturk E, Kozak O, Tufan T (2008) Lightning strike: an unusual etiology of gastric perforation. Am J Emerg Med 26:966.e5–966.e7

Kleinschmidt-DeMasters BK (1995) Neuropathology of lightning-strike injuries. Semin Neurol 15:323–328

Kleiter I, Luerding R, Diendorfer G, Rek H, Bogdahn U, Schalke B (2007) A lightning strike to the head causing a visual cortex defect with simple and complex visual hallucinations. J Neurol Neurosurg Psychiatry 78:423–426

Kotagel S, Rawlings CA, Chen S, Burris G, Nouri S (1982) Neurologic, psychiatric and cardiovascular complications in children struck by lightning. Pediatrics 70:190–192

Krauland W (1951) Schäden und Todesfälle durch Blitzschlag. Dtsch Zeitschr Gerichtl Med 40:298–312

Krause D (2004) Todesfälle durch Blitzeinwirkung. In: Brinkmann B, Madea B (eds) Handbuch gerichtliche Medizin. vol 1. Springer, Berlin, pp 835–837

Kravitz H, Wassermann MJ, Valaitis J, Anzinger RE, Naidu SH (1977) Lightning injury: management of a case with ten-day survival. Am J Dis Child 131:413–415

Kundt G, Krentz H, Glass Ä (2012) Epidemiologie und medizinische Biometrie. 7th edn. Shaker, Aachen

Kupfer J, Funke K, Erkens R (1987) Elektrischer Strom als Unfallursache, 1st edn. Tribüne, Berlin

Langerhans P (1862) Zwei Fälle von Blitzschlag. Arch Path Anat Physiol Klin Med 24:200–201

Lifschultz BD, Donoghue ER (1993a) Deaths caused by lightning. J Forensic Sci 38:353–358

Lifschultz BD, Donoghue ER (1993b) Electrical and lightning injuries. In: Spitz WU (ed) Medicolegal investigation of death. Thomas Books, Springfield, pp 516–527

Mann H, Kozic Z, Boulos MI (1983) CT of lightning injury. Am J Neuroradiol 4:976–977

Mary AK, Gomes C (2012) Lightning accidents in Uganda. International conference on lightning protection, Vienna, September 2012, Volume 978-1-4673-1898-3

McCrady-Kahn VL, Kahn AM (1981) Lightning burns. West J Med 134:215–219

Mills B, Unrau D, Parkinson C, Jones B, Yessis J, Spring K (2006) Striking back: an assessment of lightning-related fatality and injury risk in Canada. http://www.biology.ualberta.ca/facilities/safety/uploads/PDF/Lightning-relatedinjuriesandfatalitiesinCanada_FINAL-TECHNICAL_1-September-06.pdf. Accessed: 3 Jan 2023.
Möhle F, Preuss J, Madea B, Doberentz E (2015) Vier Tage überlebter Blitzschlag nach zunächst erfolgreicher Reanimation. Rechtsmedizin 25:561–565
Muehlberger T, Vogt PM, Munster AM (2001) The long-term consequences of lightning injuries. Burns 27:829–833
Murty OP (2007) Dramatic lightning injury with exit wound. J Forensic Leg Med 14:225–227
Murty OP (2009) Lightning fatality with blast, flame, heat and current effects: a macroscopic and microscopic view. J Forensic Leg Med 16:162–167
Mutter E, Langley A (2019) Cutaneous Lichtenberg figures from lightning strike. CMAJ 191:E260
Myers GJ, Colgan MT, Van Dyke DH (1977) Lightning-strike disaster among children. JAMA 238:1045–1046
Navarrete N, Rodriguez N (2016) Epidemiologic charakteristics of death by burn injury from 2000 to 2009 in Colombia, South America: a population-based study. Burns Trauma 4:8
Navarrete-Aldana N, Cooper MA, Holle RL (2014) Lightning fatalities in Colombia from 2000 to 2009. Nat Hazards 74:1349–1362
Offiah C, Heran M, Graeb D (2007) Lightning strike: a rare cause of bilateral ossicular disruption. Am J Neurorad 28:974–975
Ohashi M, Hosoda Y, Fujishiro Y, Tuyuki A, Kikuchi K, Obara H, Kitagawa N, Ishikawa T (2001) Lightning injury as a blast injury of skull, brain and visceral lesions: clinical and experimental evidences. Keio J Med 50:257–262
Oruc M, Dündar AS, Samdanci ET, Celbis O (2023) A 9-year retrospective review of lightning deaths from the eastern Anatolian region of Turkey. Forensic Sci Med Pathol 19:139–145
O'Keefe Gatewood M, Zane RD (2004) Lightning injuries. Emerg Med Clin North Am 22:369–403
Pakiam JE, Chao TC, Chia J (1981) Lightning fatalities in Singapore. Meteor Mag 110:175–187
Penning R (2006) Rechtsmedizin systematisch. UNI-MED, Bremen
Perper JA (1976) Electrical injuries. Leg Med Annu 77:135–143
Peters G (1956) Über Gehirnveränderungen nach tödlichem Blitzschlag. Dtsch Z Ges Gerichtl Med 44:743–753
Peters WJ (1983) Lightning injury. Can Med Assoc J 128:148–150
Pollak S (2000) Verkennung von tödlichen Hochspannungs- und Blitzunfällen. Arch Kriminol 206:168–179
Pollak S (2007) Elektrotraumen, Blitzschlag. In: Madea B (ed) Praxis Rechtsmedizin. 2nd edn. Springer, Berlin, pp 190–196
Pollak S, Thierauf A (2015) Elektrotraumen, Blitzschlag. In: Madea B (ed) Rechtsmedizin. 3rd edn. Springer, Berlin, pp 324–332
Pollak S, Stellwag-Carion C, Binder R (1988) Zur Pathomorphologie tödlicher Blitzunfälle. In: Bauer G (ed) Gerichtsmedizin—Festschrift für Wilhelm Holczabek. Deuticke, Wien, pp 139–153
Proportionen der Weltbevölkerung (2023) Bevölkerungszunahme in Deutschland 1950 bis 2000. http://www.pdwb.de/deu50-00.htm. Accessed: 3 Jan 2023.
Pschyrembel W (2020) Klinisches Wörterbuch, 286th edn. De Gruyter, Berlin
Puchstein S (2016) Zur Letalität von Blitzunfällen. Med Diss. Universität Rostock, Rostock
Püschel K, Kalka R, Schulz F, Zack F (2009) Tod durch Blitzschlag—Fahrrad als "(Faraday'sche) Falle". Rechtsmedizin 19:102–104

Raga GB, de la Parra MG, Kucienska B (2014) Deaths by lightning in Mexico (1979–2011): threat or vulnerability? Weather Clim Soc 6:434–444
Rakov VA, Uman MA (2006) Lightning physics and effects. Cambridge University Press, Cambridge
Reimann W, Prokop O (1980) Vademecum Gerichtsmedizin, 3rd edn. Volk und Gesundheit, Berlin
Resnik BI, Wetli CV (1996) Lichtenberg figures. Am J Forensic Med Pathol 17:99–102
Ritenour AE, Morton MJ, McManus JG, Barillo DJ, Cancio LC (2008) Lightning injury: a review. Burns 34:585–594
Rothschild MA (2009) Probleme bei der ärztlichen Leichenschau. Sicht der niedergelassenen Ärzte, der Klinikärzte, der Notärzte und der Polizei. Rechtsmedizin 19:407–412
Saleem R, Riyaz N, Anupama MA (2013) Gold granuloma in a beaded pattern due to lightning strike: a unique presentation. Indian J Dermatol Venereol Leprol 79:430–431
Sanford A, Gamelli RL (2014) Lightning and thermal injuries. Handb Clin Neurol 120:981–986
Schaidt G (1977) Spuren an Kleidungsstücken beim Blitzunfall. Arch Kriminol 159:93–96
Schniers E (2005) Schädigungen und Tod nach Blitzschlag—eine Synopsis aus rechtsmedizinischer Sicht. Med Diss. Universität Rostock, Rostock
Schroeder M (1991) Fractals, chaos, power laws—minutes from an infinite paradise. Freeman, New York
Schwab M, Wiegand H, Bentsen P, Hochrein H (1989) Infarkt-EKG nach Blitzunfall. Z Kardiol 78:611–614
Schwerd W (1992) Rechtsmedizin. Deutscher Ärzte-Verlag, Köln
Sellier K (1975) Schäden und Tod durch Elektrizität. In: Mueller B (ed) Gerichtliche Medizin. 2nd edn. Teil 1. Springer, Berlin, pp 538–563
Skan DA (1949) Death from lightning-stroke, with multiple injuries. Br Med J 1:666
Sleihwah A, Baker J, Gowers C, Elsom DM, Rashid A (2018) Lightning injuries in Northern Ireland. Ulster Med J 87:168–172
Spaar FW (1955) Hirnbefund nach Tod durch Blitzschlag. Virchows Arch 326:732–747
Statistisches Bundesamt Deutschland (2020) Gestorbene an Unfall durch Blitzschlag. Statistisches Bundesamt Deutschland, Zweigstelle Bonn
Stoff M, Baumgärtner W, Wohlsein P (2020) Blitzschlag auf der Pferdeweide—eine diagnostische Herausforderung?! Tierarztl Prax/G 48:268–274
Strasser EJ, Davis RM, Menchey MJ (1977) Lightning injuries. J Trauma 17:315–319
Ströhle M, Wallner B, Lanthaler M, Rauch S, Brugger H, Paal P (2018) Lightning accidents in the Austrian alps—a 10-year retrospective nationwide analysis. Scand J Trauma Resusc Emerg Med 26:74
Stütz N, Weiss D, Reichert B (2006) Verletzungen durch Blitzschlag. Unfallchirurg 109:495–498
Tadler M, Rüegg E, Niquille M, Gencer B, Gautschi OP, Pittet-Cuénod B, Modarressi A (2017) Multi-organ injuries due to a lightning strike: a case report highlighting the importance of a multi-disciplinary approach. Case Reports Plast Surg Hand Surg 4:1–4
Thacker MF, Lee R, Sabogal RI, Henderson A (2008) Overview of deaths associated with natural events, United States, 1979–2004. Disasters 32:303–325
Tribble CG, Persing JA, Morgan RF, Kenney JG, Edlich RF (1985) Lightning injuries. Compr Ther 11:32–40
Uman MA (1986) All about lightning. Dover Publications, New York
Uman MA (2008) The art and science of lightning protection. Cambridge University Press, Cambridge
Ventura F, Barranco R, Bonsignore A, De Stefano F (2017) A unusual lightning death in an indoor setting. A case report. Am J Forensic Med Pathol 38:1–4

Walsh KM, Cooper MA, Holle R, Rakov VA, Roeder WP, Ryan M (2013) National athletic trainers' association safety for athletics and recreation. J Athl Train 48:258–270

Wankhede AG (2022) A unique case of direct lightning strike. J Forensic Sci 67:1288–1293

Weimann W, Prokop O (1963) Atlas der gerichtlichen Medizin. Volk und Gesundheit, Berlin

Wetli CV (1996) Keraunopathology. An analysis of 45 fatalities. Am J Forensic Med Pathol 17:89–98

Whitcomb D, Martinez JA, Daberkow D (2002) Lightning injuries. South Med J 95:1331–1334

World Health Organisation (2022) International classification of diseases and related health problems (ICD). 10. Revision. WHO, Genf

Zack F, Büttner A (2016) Rechtsmedizinische Aspekte der Lichtenberg-Figuren nach Blitzschlag. Rechtsmedizin 26:425–428

Zack F, Büttner A (2020) Blitzunfall. Teil 2: Pathophysiologische und diagnostische Aspekte bei tödlichen Ereignissen. Rechtsmedizin 30:345–356

Zack F, Hammer U, Klett I, Wegener R (1997) Myocardial injury due to lightning. Int J Legal Med 110:326–328

Zack F, Rummel J, Püschel K (2009) Blitzschläge auf Fußballplätzen. Eine unterschätzte Gefahr. Rechtsmedizin 19:77–82

Zack F, Rammelsberg JO, Graf B, Büttner A (2010) Tod durch Blitzschlag—und wieder unter einem Baum. Rechtsmedizin 20:108–110

Zack F, Raphael T, Kupfer J, Jokuszies A, Vogt PM, Büttner A, Püschel K, Schalke B, Todt M, Dettmeyer R (2013) Vier Todesopfer nach einem Blitzunfall auf einem Golfplatz. Rechtsmedizin 23:114–118

Zack F, Puchstein S, Büttner A (2016) Letalität von Blitzunfällen. Rechtsmedizin 26:9–11

Zack F, Kaden A, Riepenhausen S, Rentsch D, Kegler R, Büttner A (2017) Fehler bei der Ausstellung der Todesbescheinigung. Eine Analyse von 10.000 Sterbefällen aus Mecklenburg. Rechtsmedizin 27:516–527

Zack F, Schau H, Dalchow A, Rock M, Blaas V, Büttner A (2020) Lesions and characteristic injury patterns caused by high-voltage fault arcs. Int J Legal Med 134:1353–1359

Zimmermann C, Cooper MA, Holle RL (2002) Lightning safety guidelines. Ann Emerg Med 39:665–670

8 Prevention

Particularly due to the possibilities that a person can die from a lightning strike accident or can show persistent late effects, prevention is always better than any therapy. In this context, extensive basic knowledge and its application are at the center of prevention.

8.1 Location-dependent Risk

With the exception of the regions around the North and South Poles, thunderstorms are ubiquitous meteorological events on Earth that make every human a potential victim of a lightning strike. Even though some literature sources suggest that houses and closed vehicles as Faraday cages are safe places, specific accidents show that perhaps with the exception of the Arctic and Antarctic, there are no absolutely safe places for injuries from a lightning strike for humans on Earth (Angerer et al. 2009; Blanco-Pampin et al. 1997; Holle 2010; Uman 2008). However, there are areas that are safer than others (Holle et al. 1999; Rakov and Uman 2006). It is undisputed in the technical literature that most accidents involving lightning strikes with personal injury occur outdoors (Cooper and Holle 2019). Retrospective studies show that there are a number of places or activities where humans are particularly at risk (Harms 1956; Cherington 2001; Eriksson and Örnehult 1988).

> **Note** Even houses and closed vehicles are not absolutely safe places. However, they are safer than other areas.

F. Zack, *Accidents Caused by Lightning Strikes*,
https://doi.org/10.1007/978-3-662-71066-1_8

Places where accidents involving lightning strikes with personal injury occur frequently

- Under a freestanding tree, rows of trees or groups of trees
- On a field, a meadow or pasture
- On football, golf courses and other large open areas
- In the mountains
- At or on waters
- On rooftops
- In tents

Activities during which a person is particularly at risk of suffering a lightning strike

- Unprotected work in agriculture
- Hikingand mountaineering
- Cycling
- Playing golf or football outdoors
- Attending open-air events
- Fishing
- Camping
- Working on roofs
- Performing military service outdoors

The mere existence of the phenomenon "bolt from the blue" and the impossibility, despite all technical advances, for meteorologists to accurately predict the locations of lightning strikes in stormy weather conditions, means that there can be no absolute avoidance of lightning accidents for people in the future (Blumenthal 2022; Cherington et al. 1997; Kleiter et al. 2007). However, the significant decrease in fatal events, which has been observed for about 70 years, particularly in Europe and North America, shows that people are on the right track in terms of avoiding lethal accidents caused by lightning strikes. The causes for this regression appear to be diverse (Cooper and Holle 2019; Schniers 2005).

Factors that are presumably co-responsible for the decline in the number of lethal accidents caused by lightning strikes, particularly in Europe and North America, in recent decades

- Decrease in the number of unprotected workers in agriculture
- Increase in the approvals of enclosed vehicles

- Increase in the number of enclosed buildings
- Increase in knowledge about proper behavior during thunderstorms
- Increase in media presence with explanations, weather reports, and warnings
- Faster and improved medical treatment

Since no one can predict after a lightning strike accident whether the victim will be slightly, moderately, severely, or fatally injured, prevention always comes first (Cooper et al. 2017; Blumenthal 2021).

8.2 Preventive Measures

Apparently also due to the significantly larger number of lightning accidents with injured and killed persons per nation, particularly physicians from the USA have made contributions to the topic of prevention in recent decades. In doing so, the doctors have cooperated with scientists from numerous other fields (Cooper et al. 1999, 2017; Hunt et al. 2020; Zimmermann et al. 2002).

In Germany, where less than 10 people per year have died from lightning strikes for about three decades, the Committee for Lightning Protection and Lightning Research of the Association for Electrical, Electronic and Information Technologies has primarily taken care of the prevention of lightning accidents. In the German-speaking neighboring countries, Electrosuisse and the Austrian Association for Electrical Engineering have taken on this task. The focus here is on educating the population and protecting buildings (Heidler and Stimper 2009; Association for Electrical, Electronic and Information Technologies et al. 2023).

8.2.1 Basic Knowledge

In most lightning strike accidents involving personal injury, only one victim is injured. The possibility of a mass casualty event exists where crowds gather, for example at folk festivals, sports events, or open-air concerts. Personal behavior to avoid accidents caused by lightning strikes should always be proactive. Reacting to lightning strikes in the immediate vicinity is always the worse solution.

Widespread basic knowledge is important in order to make the right decisions during the dangerous times when a lightning strike threatens.

The high relevance of prevention arises inevitably from the sometimes far-reaching consequences of lightning strike injuries (see Chaps. 1 and 4–7). The key to high safety lies in individual education and the practical implementation of knowledge. Results from the National Lightning Data Network in the USA about cloud-to-ground lightning revealed that deaths and injuries from lightning strikes generally occur in equal parts before, during, and after the strongest lightning activity in a thunderstorm (Holle et al. 1998; Lengyel et al. 2005). Weak thunderstorms claim at least as many victims as moderate or strong ones (Holle 1993). A study by Lengyel et al. (2005) found that almost half of the victims of lightning strikes had been sufficiently warned beforehand to take safety precautions in time. In July 2014, accidents occurred in Rocky Mountains National Park (USA) on two consecutive days during storms with low lightning rates, injuring a total of 12 people, two of whom died. The distance between the two accident sites was 2.8 km (Hodanish et al. 2015).

An interdisciplinary group of lightning protection experts developed in the USA in 1998 new guidelines, as these had not been meaningfully adapted for several decades (Holle et al. 1999; Zimmermann et al. 2002). The development of national lightning detection networks and the availability of other meteorological datasets had led to a fundamental rethink of existing guidelines. Since 1998, most guidelines have been evaluated and further adapted. At the current time, most recommendations from before 1998 are considered to be based on erroneous assumptions and are obsolete (Cooper et al. 2017).

8.2.2 Prevention through Planning

For a person who follows the weather report and observes the sky, a lightning strike rarely appears so suddenly that no precautions could be taken to minimize the risk. Thunderstorms need at least 10 minutes to develop or move into an area. An unpleasant surprise can be avoided by a series of steps. A safety plan includes knowing the safest place and estimating how far in advance measures should be taken to reach this place.

Individuals should inquire about weather forecasts and lightning information services before working outdoors or taking a recreational trip. If thunderstorms are predicted for a later time of day, it is strongly recommended to keep up with updates in the media (mobile phone). It should also be taken into account that weather data are not always completely up-to-date.

Most lightning strike accidents occur in the warm season between 12 and 18 o'clock (Schniers 2005; Wetli 1996). On days with thunderstorm warnings, hikes and other outdoor activities should therefore be undertaken in the morning or be avoided. Summer heat thunderstorms can last into the evening hours. Unfortunately, this is also the time of day when recreational athletes and those seeking relaxation are often outdoors (Andrews 1995; Cooper et al. 2017).

In the open nature or wilderness, outside of a building or a fully enclosed vehicle with a metal roof, there is no relative safety from a lightning strike.

The two approaches to lightning protection in the open nature consist of accepting that there is a risk of lightning and avoiding this risk from the outset.

Once a hike or the ascent of a mountain is underway, one should pay attention to developing cloud formations that indicate future lightning, stop the hike or ascent, and take safety precautions if necessary (Cooper et al. 2017).

8.2.3 Rules for an Approaching Thunderstorm

Developing cumulonimbus clouds, which are taller than they are wide, are usually the first signs of an impending thunderstorm (Fig. 8.1). Everyone should then pay more attention to lightning than to rain. Approximately 10% of all cloud-to-ground lightning strikes occur without precipitation at the ground, so waiting for rain does not provide protection from lightning strikes when a thunderstorm is approaching. Thunder can be heard up to a distance of 16 km under quiet conditions, but not nearly as far with ambient noises or inside a building. The simplest rule at the start of a thunderstorm is: *"When thunder roars, go indoors"* (Roeder et al. 2003). This rule eliminates any debate about when the right time to act has come. Although there may be overwarnings due to distant lightning strikes that may not reach a location, this is an effective and simple way to

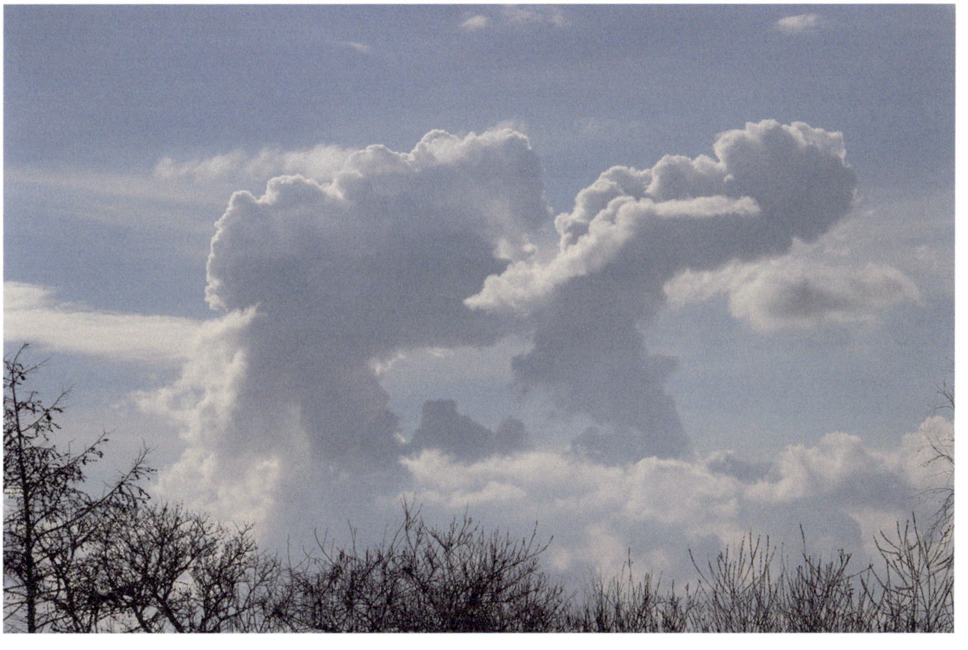

Fig. 8.1 Two typical cumulonimbus clouds in March 2023 over Mecklenburg-Western Pomerania (Germany) as a sign of a developing thunderstorm. (Own illustration)

deal with the risk of lightning. A rule with a somewhat more objective approach is the 30-30 rule, which was developed in 1998 as part of the development of new lightning protection guidelines by an interdisciplinary team of experts in the USA (Cooper et al. 1999; Holle et al. 1999; Zaffren et al. 2005; Zimmermann et al. 2002). The first number 30 refers to the time in seconds between seeing a flash of lightning and hearing the thunder of the lightning. If the interval from the flash to the thunder is 30 s or less, people are at risk from lightning strikes and should actively seek the safest possible place. Measured or even counted 30 s indicate that a lightning strike has occurred no more than 10 km from the location of this person, assuming a speed of sound of 343 m/s. Ten kilometers cover about 80% of all subsequent cloud-to-ground lightning strikes of a thunderstorm. Variations of the 30-s rule are often used at military and civilian airports for radii between 8 and 16 km, where validated cloud-to-ground lightning detection systems are used. In such situations, too many warnings from a large radius around a point can lead to a lack of trust in the method, while too small a radius can overlook too many thunderstorms and thus potentially dangerous lightning strikes (Cooper et al. 2017).

8.2.4 Rules at the End of a Thunderstorm

At the end of a thunderstorm, the risk of lightning should not be underestimated, as during this period just as many people are killed or injured by lightning strikes as at the beginning or in the middle of a thunderstorm. A number of people die each year, for example, because they impatiently leave the relatively safe area of a house too early and go outside (Cooper et al. 2017). The second number 30 of the 30-30 rule states that one should wait 30 minutes after perceiving the last flash of lightning or thunder before going outside again (Cooper et al. 1999; Holle et al. 1999; Zimmermann et al. 2002). At night, lightning can be visible up to 80 km away in high thunderstorms. These are not dangerous for the observer unless the lightning channel itself is visible until it reaches the ground (Cooper et al. 2017).

Since the guidelines of 1998, it has been found that the time span of 30 minutes was relatively generous, as in most situations the risk of lightning was only considered minimal after 15 minutes. Therefore, this recommendation was modified. A single person or even small groups can already leave the relatively safe place 15 minutes after the last flash of lightning or thunder and stay nearby, so that this can be reached again in the shortest possible time if the thunderstorm returns. For large groups of people and crowds, the initially recommended 30 minutes still apply.

There are also exceptions to the 30-30 rule, for example, when an extensive, high-altitude thunderstorm lingers over a place for hours. Then, *"safety first"* should always apply (Cooper et al. 2017).

8.2.5 Relatively Safe Places

There are two relatively safe places where one can protect oneself from a lightning strike: in a large, solid, completed building with closed windows and doors, and in a closed vehicle with a metal body or at least a metal roof.

If people are caught outside in a thunderstorm, taking shelter under a bridge may also offer some protection.

8.2.5.1 Buildings

Large buildings where people live and work are relatively lightning-proof in developed countries. Although houses are also directly hit by lightning strikes, deaths in them are extremely rare, especially considering how much time people spend in them. A study from the USA recorded a total of 31 deaths from lightning strikes that occurred in houses nationwide over a 17-year period (1992–2008). Children and older people, as well as people with disabilities who were obviously unable to leave the apartment in time in the event of a fire caused by a lightning strike, were particularly affected. There were no deaths in schools, train stations, or other large public buildings. As a result, it can be assumed that the danger during a thunderstorm for people in enclosed buildings without lightning protection equipment is most likely to come from open fire (Holle 2010).

The protection in modern buildings for people and inventory is best ensured by an external and internal lightning protection system. The external system serves to catch a lightning strike before it hits the building, to conduct the current to the ground, and to distribute the current in the ground (Figs. 8.2 and 8.3).

The internal lightning protection system, on the other hand, is designed to prevent dangerous sparking within the facility to be protected (Heidler and Stimper 2009). Contact with corded telephones and other electrical devices connected to a socket can lead to severe injuries, as can staying near open windows or doors, and should therefore be avoided (Andrews 1992; Cooper et al. 2017).

In Germany, there is no general obligation to install an external lightning protection system. The external system is only required for certain structures after an assessment of the building-related risk. This particularly applies to public buildings such as clinics, schools, or theaters, high-rise buildings, particularly high and exposed houses, older houses with roofs made of easily flammable materials such as reeds or wood, as well as historical buildings. The corresponding regulations can be found, among other things, in the building regulations of the federal states.

Fundamentally unsafe indoor areas are open objects such as shelters, huts, stops, construction sites, etc. Such places must be abandoned in favor of a larger building or a safe vehicle. Tents only offer protection against rain, but not against lightning strikes (Carte et al. 2002; Lindfort et al. 2017; Mutter and Langley 2019; van Zomeren et al. 1998; Zack et al. 1997). In less developed countries, homes and workplaces can be thatched huts, which also offer no protection against lightning strikes, as they are usually not grounded and are made of non-conductive material (Holle 2010).

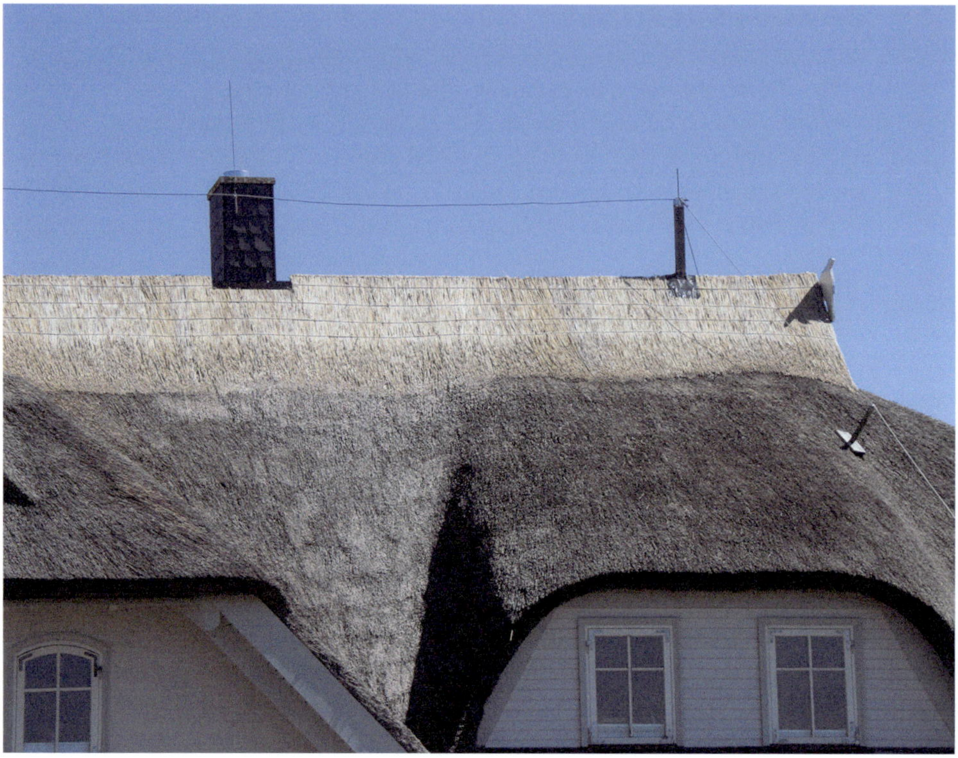

Fig. 8.2 Parts of the external lightning protection system with a catching device (e.g., vertical metal rod on the chimney) and a discharge device. (Own illustration)

8.2.5.2 Vehicles

Fully enclosed vehicles with a metal roof offer as a Faraday cage good protection against electric current during a lightning strike and should be used as relatively safe places when no buildings are nearby. In addition to cars with the described conditions, cabins of construction machinery, railway wagons or metal cabins of cable cars also offer this protection (Electrosuisse 2019; Association of Electrical Engineering Electronics Information Technology et al. 2023).

In the event of a direct hit on the vehicle, however, occupants can be injured by a blast trauma or a blinding effect of the lightning channel. There is a documented case in the literature where an older man drove into oncoming traffic with his car after a lightning strike nearby and died from the consequences of the accident. No fatalities due to the transfer of electrical energy into the vehicle have been reported so far. The damage to struck vehicles ranges from evaporated antennas to engine failures to electrical fires (Angerer et al. 2009; Cooper et al. 2017). In the event of a direct hit on a vehicle with

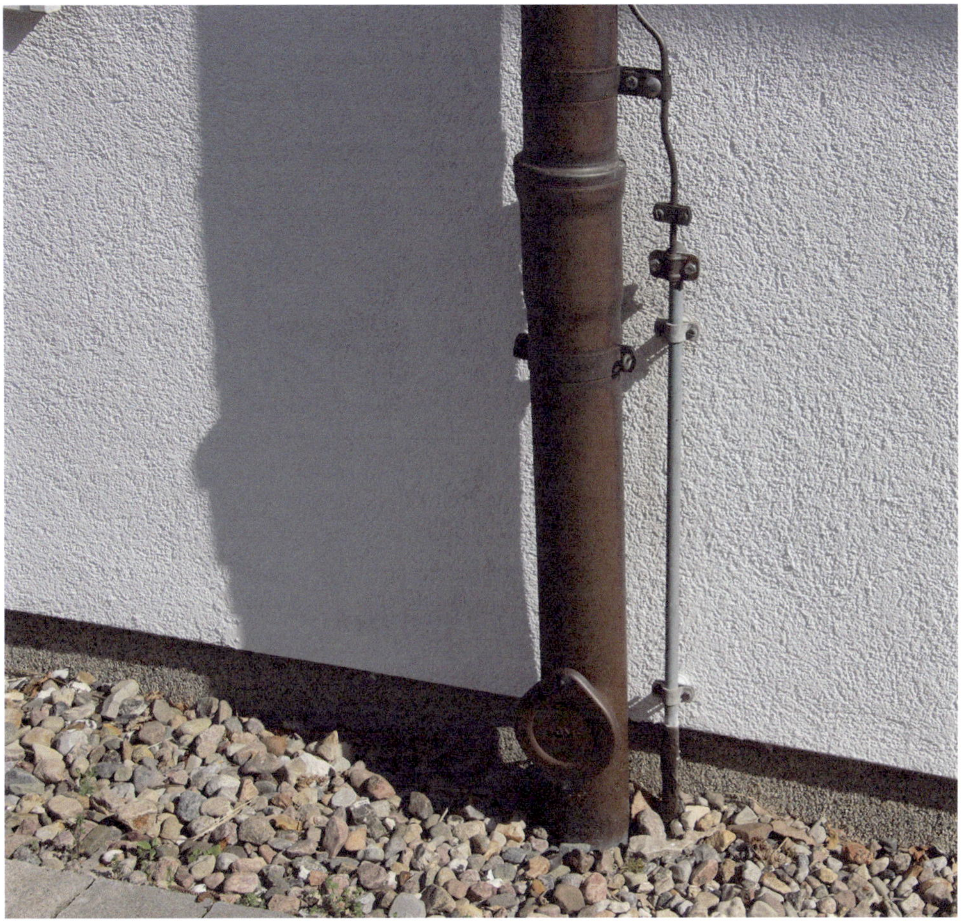

Fig. 8.3 The grounding system next to a copper downpipe as part of the external lightning protection system. (Own illustration)

a metal body or metal roof, the electrical energy is discharged to the earth via the outer shell with a subsequent arc. In connection with staying in or on a vehicle, a person can also be injured when getting in or out, either by a direct hit or by step voltage.

Unsafe vehicles that do not represent a Faraday cage include convertibles with fabric roofs, vehicles without a metal body, golf carts, and vehicles with open sides (Cooper et al. 2017; Zimmermann et al. 2002).

8.2.5.3 Bridges

Harms (1956) found in an evaluation of 267 accidents caused by lightning strikes with 173 fatalities and 231 injured persons in Germany in the period from 1950–1955 no case that occurred under a bridge. He concluded from this that in addition to buildings and vehicles, bridge passages should also be sought when a thunderstorm is approaching. Also, in our own research in the medical literature, no accident under a bridge with one or more fatalities has been found so far. An inquiry to the head of the department of lightning and surge protection at the Technical University of Ilmenau (Germany) on this topic revealed that he also has no knowledge of lightning strike accidents with the injury of a person while staying under bridges. The location can possibly only protect against an accident by a direct hit. When staying under a bridge in case of thunderstorm danger, it is important to keep a few meters distance from the ends, the supports or the masts. The bridge above the person creates a protective space, as a lightning bolt growing from the cloud is most likely to strike the bridge and can only hit a person below the bridge with very low probability, rather coming from the side. To avoid further types of lightning effects (see Chap. 4) caused by the lightning currents flowing over the bridge construction and the earth-connected supports after a strike into the bridge, the distance of the person seeking protection to all parts of the bridge, also upwards, should be a few meters. This idea can be derived from the principles of lightning protection of buildings (M. Rock, personal communication, January 8, 2023).

Relevance for Prevention

- There is no absolute safety from accidents caused by lightning strikes in the populated latitudes of the earth.
- Relatively safe places are large, solid, completed buildings with closed doors and windows, as well as closed vehicles with a metal body or at least a metal roof.
- The consequences of a lightning strike for a person's health are unpredictable.
- Since no one can predict whether a victim will be lightly, moderately, severely, or fatally injured after a lightning strike accident, prevention is better than any therapy.
- Particularly when planning outdoor activities, weather forecasts should be taken into account and considered.
- Modern communication possibilities (e.g., mobile phones) should be included in prevention in case of potential thunderstorm danger.
- Everyone should know the 30-30 rule and behave accordingly.

References

Andrews CJ (1992) Telephon related lightning injury. Med J Australia 157:823–828

Andrews CJ (1995) Keraunomedicine: A discipline come of age. Ann Emerg Med 25:543–545

Angerer F, Hoppe U, Schick B (2009) Blitzeinschlag in einen PKW mit Schädigung des Hörorgans. HNO 57:1081–1084

Blanco-Pampin JM, Suarez-Penaranda JM, Rico-Boquete R, Concheira-Carro L (1997) An unusual case of death by lightning. J Forensic Sci 42:942–944

Blumenthal R (2021) Injuries and deaths from lightning. J Clin Pathol 74:279–284

Blumenthal R (2022) Lightning metallization injury. Am J Forensic Med Pathol 43:e93–e95

Carte AE, Anderson RB, Cooper MA (2002) A large group of children struck by lightning. Ann Emerg Med 39:665–670

Cherington M (2001) Lightning injuries in sports: situations to avoid. Sports Med 31:301–308

Cherington M, Krider EP, Yarnell PR, Breed DW (1997) A bolt from the blue: lightning strike to the head. Neurology 48:683–686

Cooper MA, Holle RL (2019) Reducing lightning injuries worldwide. Springer, Cham

Cooper MA, Holle RL, Lopez R (1999) Recommendations for lightning safety. JAMA 282:1132–1133

Cooper MA, Andrews CJ, Holle RL, Blumenthal R, Navarette-Aldana N (2017) Lightning-related injuries and safety. In: Auerbach P, Cushing T, Harris N (Eds) Auerbach's wilderness medicine. 7th edn. Elsevier, Philadelphia, pp 71–117

Electrosuisse (2019) Blitze. So können Sie sich schützen. https://www.electrosuisse.ch/wp-content/uploads/2019/03/Electrosuisse_Blitzeschutz_Broschuere.pdf. Accessed: 22. March 2023

Eriksson A, Örnehult L (1988) Death by lightning. Am J Forensic Med Pathol 9:295–300

Harms W (1956) Personenblitzschäden. Elektromedizin 1:153–158

Heidler F, Stimper K (2009) Blitz und Blitzschutz. VDE, Berlin Offenbach

Hodanish S, Wolyn P, Mozley K (2015) Meteorological analysis of the Rocky Mountain National Park lightning fatalities of 11 and 12 July, 2014. https://www.weather.gov/media/pub/pdf/Lightning/PDFs/RMNP_fatalities_AMS2015_MOD.pdf. Accessed: 12 Dec 2022

Holle RL (1993) The local meteorological environment of lightning casualities in central Florida. 17th Conference on severe local storms. 4.–8. Oktober, St. Louis, Missouri

Holle RL (2010) Lightning-caused casualities in and near dwellings and other buildings. https://www.vaisala.com/sites/default/files/documents/9.Holle-Lightning-Caused.pdf. Accessed: 14 Dec 2022

Holle RL, Lopez RE, Zimmermann C (1999) Update recommendations for lightning safety—1998. Bull Am Meteor Soc 80:2035–2041

Hunt HGP, Blumenthal R, Nixon KJ, Gomes C (2020) A multidisciplinary forensic analysis of two lightning deaths observed in South Africa. Int J Disaster Risk Reduct 51:101814

Kleiter I, Luerding R, Dienhofer G, Rek H, Bogdahn U, Schalke B (2007) A lightning strike to the head causing a visual cortex defect with simple and complex visual hallucinations. J Neurol Neurosurg Psychiatry 78:423–426

Lengyel M, Brooks H, Holle RL (2005) Lightning casualities and their proximity to surrounding cloud-to-ground lightning casuality worldwide. 14th Symposium on education, 8.–14. Januar, San Diego, California

Lindfort A, Vuola J, Kankuri E (2017) Resuscitated unconscious male: Lichtenberg's sign lightning the way. Intensive Care Med 43:1148–1149
Mutter E, Langley A (2019) Cutaneous Lichtenberg figures from lightning strike. CMAJ 191:E260
Rakov VA, Uman MA (2006) Lightning. Physics and effects. Cambridge University Press, Cambridge New York Melbourne Madrid Cape Town Singapore Sao Paulo
Roeder WP, Cooper MA, Holle RL (2003) Updated lightning recommendations for lightning safety—2002. Bull Am Met Soc 84:261–266
Schniers E (2005) Schädigung und Tod nach Blitzschlag – eine Synopsis aus rechtsmedizinischer Sicht. Med Diss. Universität Rostock, Rostock
Uman MA (2008) The art and science of lightning protection. Cambridge University Press, Cambridge New York Melbourne Madrid Kapstadt Singapur Sao Paulo Delhi
Van Zomeren AH, ten Duis HK, Minderhoud JM, Sipma M (1998) Lightning stroke and neuropsychological impairment: cases and questions. J Neurol Neurosurg Psychiatry 64:763–769
Verband der Elektrotechnik Elektronik Informationstechnik e. V., Österreichischer Verband für Elektrotechnik, Electrosuisse (2023) Vor Blitzen schützen. https://www.vor-blitzen-schuetzen.eu/de. Accessed: 22 March 2023
Wetli CW (1996) Keraunopathology. An analysis of 45 fatalities. Am J Forensic Med Pathol 17:89–98
Zack F, Hammer U, Klett I, Wegener R (1997) Myocardial injury due to lightning. Int J Legal Med 110:326–328
Zafren K, Durrer B, Herry JP, Brugger H, ICAR MEDCOM, UIAA MEDCOM, (2005) Lightning injuries: prevention and on-site treatment in mountains and remote areas. Official guidelines of the International Commission for Mountain Emergency Medicine and the Medical Commission of the International Mountaineering and Climbing Federation. Resuscitation 65:369–372
Zimmermann C, Cooper MA, Holle RL (2002) Lightning safety guidelines. Ann Emerg Med 39:660–664

MIX
Papier aus verantwortungsvollen Quellen
Paper from responsible sources
FSC® C105338
FSC
www.fsc.org

If you have any concerns about our products,
you can contact us on
ProductSafety@springernature.com

In case Publisher is established outside the EU,
the EU authorized representative is:
Springer Nature Customer Service Center GmbH
Europaplatz 3, 69115 Heidelberg, Germany

Printed by Libri Plureos GmbH
in Hamburg, Germany